# Fatigue Stability

How Energy Loss, Recovery Debt, and System Strain Shape Daily Function

Nathan Reed

PERENNIAL PUBLISHING

Published by Perennial Publishing



Paperback ISBN: 978-1-971996-60-8
Hardcover ISBN: 978-1-971996-61-5
E-book ISBN: 978-1-971996-62-2

# Contents

# Fatigue as a Stability Signal

Fatigue is one of the most familiar human experiences and one of the most consistently misinterpreted. Nearly everyone recognizes the feeling of heaviness, slowed thinking, reduced tolerance, unstable motivation, diminished output, or the sense that ordinary tasks suddenly require disproportionate effort. Yet despite how common fatigue is, the interpretation of fatigue often collapses immediately into judgment. Exhaustion becomes laziness. Reduced output becomes poor discipline. Slowed function becomes weakness, low resilience, lack of drive, or insufficient effort.

The sensation is treated as a character problem before it is treated as system information.

This interpretation shapes how fatigue is experienced long before it is understood. A person becomes tired and assumes something has failed morally rather than physiologically. The body narrows usable function, and the response is often frustration, self-criticism, denial, overcompensation, or attempts to override the signal indefinitely. Fatigue is framed as an obstacle to productivity rather than as information about the relationship between demand and available capacity.

This book approaches fatigue differently.

Fatigue Stability examines fatigue as a stability signal produced by the body under conditions of strain, recovery debt, rising system cost, narrowed support capacity, unstable fuel availability, nervous system activation, disrupted restoration, or accumulating adaptation pressure.

Fatigue is treated here not as weakness, but as communication emerging from the interaction among systems responsible for sustaining usable function across time.

The central shift is interpretive.

Fatigue becomes more understandable when viewed as information about system state rather than as evidence of personal inadequacy.

This does not mean all fatigue carries the same meaning or intensity. Human physiology fluctuates naturally. Temporary exhaustion after concentrated effort, disrupted sleep, emotional stress, travel, illness, prolonged cognitive demand, or high activity is part of normal biological function. The body continuously adjusts output according to current conditions. Capacity rises and falls. Recovery depth changes. Stress exposure changes. Fuel continuity changes. Sleep quality changes. Human systems are dynamic rather than static.

Fatigue becomes more difficult to interpret when every form of exhaustion is treated as identical.

This is part of why fatigue often feels confusing. Some fatigue appears as heaviness. Some appears as fog, irritability, reduced emotional tolerance, slowed recovery, unstable concentration, reduced drive, or delayed crashes after prolonged stress. Some fatigue emerges gradually through narrowing reserve capacity across weeks or months. Some appears sharply when thresholds are crossed after long periods of compensation underneath visible function.

The body communicates through patterns of constrained usable function rather than through one single universal sensation.

Energy Stability examined the continuity side of this relationship: how the body sustains usable output through fuel coordination, recovery, metabolic flexibility, nervous system regulation, and broader energetic continuity across time. Fatigue Stability examines the opposing pressure within the same system relationship. If energy continuity reflects the body's ability to sustain usable function, fatigue reflects the pressures narrowing, destabilizing, slowing, or reducing that function under accumulating strain.

The two are inseparable.

Usable function does not disappear randomly. The body continuously negotiates between demand and support capacity. When maintaining current output becomes increasingly expensive relative to available reserve, fatigue signals begin appearing more prominently. The body may reduce output, narrow tolerance, slow recovery, amplify warning, or enforce downshift partly because preserving stability has become more difficult under existing conditions.

Fatigue therefore belongs inside metabolic stability rather than outside it.

It is not separate from physiology and not reducible to mindset alone. Fatigue reflects the relationship between load and support capacity across time.

Load includes more than visible physical exertion. Stress load, emotional demand, cognitive pressure, uncertainty, nervous system strain, immune strain, poor sleep, glucose instability, compensation cost, transition friction, and unresolved recovery debt all increase the energetic expense required to maintain continuity. A person may appear externally inactive while internally carrying substantial regulation burden underneath persistent activation, vigilance, emotional suppression, adaptation demand, or unstable recovery.

The body responds to total system cost rather than visible effort alone.

Capacity also extends beyond simple motivation. Support capacity depends partly on restoration depth, fuel continuity, sleep-recovery translation, stress containment, nervous system flexibility, electrolyte signal integrity, and broader metabolic coordination. The body continuously adjusts usable output according to how much reserve remains available to absorb demand without excessive destabilization.

Fatigue appears partly when this relationship narrows.

The important distinction is that fatigue is not identical to failure. The body reducing output under strain is not inherently irrational or defective. Earlier forms of compensation may preserve visible function temporarily through urgency, adrenaline, caffeine, obligation, routine, or narrowed focus. But compensation increases system cost when restoration repeatedly falls short of demand underneath ongoing output.

The resulting exhaustion often becomes visible later through crashes, heaviness, reduced tolerance, slowed recovery, emotional narrowing, or unstable function.

Fatigue therefore is not simply the absence of energy. It is frequently the signal that sustaining current output has become increasingly expensive relative to available support capacity.

This distinction changes the meaning of reduced function entirely.

The body is not merely becoming "unmotivated." It may be protecting remaining stability margin under conditions of accumulating strain. Downshift, reduced drive, slowed movement, narrowed concentration, or emotional exhaustion often represent protective reductions rather than moral collapse. The system continuously attempts to preserve continuity under changing conditions.

Fatigue is part of that protective communication.

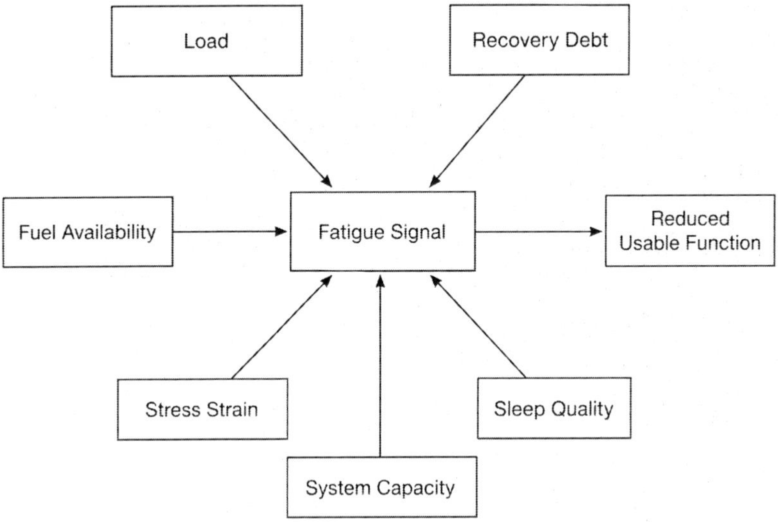


**[Figure 1: Fatigue as a Stability Signal]**

The relationships represented here clarify why fatigue is better understood as a systems signal rather than a personal verdict. Load, recovery debt, fuel availability, stress strain, sleep quality, and broader system capacity all influence the intensity and visibility of fatigue signals across time. As these pressures interact, usable function may narrow, slow, destabilize, or become more expensive to sustain. Fatigue emerges not as random weakness, but as information about the body's current relationship between demand and support capacity.

This perspective also explains why fatigue should not be ignored indefinitely. Signals exist because they communicate changing system conditions. Overriding exhaustion repeatedly through compensation, activation, urgency, or self-judgment often increases regulation cost underneath continued output. Recovery debt accumulates quietly. Thresholds narrow. Stress signaling remains elevated. Restoration becomes less efficient. The body spends increasing resources preserving continuity while usable reserve gradually decreases.

Fatigue eventually becomes more difficult to suppress because the underlying system pressure continues rising.

At the same time, fatigue should not become identity. Human physiology fluctuates continuously. Temporary exhaustion does not automatically define the individual experiencing it. The body's current state is not equivalent to permanent character. Fatigue can be meaningful without becoming catastrophic.

This distinction matters because many people oscillate between dismissal and over-identification. One person ignores exhaustion entirely and interprets every signal as weakness to overcome. Another interprets every fluctuation as evidence of irreversible dysfunction. Both interpretations distort the signal.

Fatigue is neither meaningless nor absolute.

The goal of this book is therefore not prescription, optimization, or performance enhancement. It is interpretation. The objective is to understand fatigue structurally rather than morally. Human physiology becomes more understandable when exhaustion is viewed through load, capacity, recovery debt, fuel continuity, stress strain, sleep quality, compensation cost, and broader stability relationships rather than through shame or simplistic motivation narratives alone.

This framework also preserves appropriate caution. Severe, persistent, worsening, unusual, or unexplained fatigue should not be dismissed casually. Human physiology is complex, and significant exhaustion deserves attention rather than automatic normalization.

The important shift remains interpretive rather than diagnostic.

Fatigue becomes useful when it is understood as information emerging from system relationships rather than as evidence of personal failure. The body continuously communicates through usable function, reduced tolerance, slowed recovery, heaviness, crashes, fog, and downshift because maintaining stability under current conditions carries real physiological cost.

The signal is attempting to describe the state of the system.

And once fatigue is viewed through that lens, a different question begins emerging underneath the exhaustion itself. The important issue is no longer simply whether fatigue exists. The important issue becomes what the fatigue signal is revealing about load, capacity, recovery debt, and the body's current ability to sustain usable function across time.

# Signal Mechanism

Fatigue is one of the most familiar human experiences and one of the most frequently misinterpreted. It is felt directly, often daily, and usually with enough immediacy that interpretation occurs before analysis. A person wakes exhausted after sleeping, loses usable function in the middle of the afternoon, feels mentally slowed under prolonged stress, or notices that ordinary tasks suddenly require disproportionate effort. The experience is uncomfortable, visible, disruptive, and difficult to separate from identity. Because of this, fatigue is often interpreted morally before it is interpreted physiologically.

The interpretation usually happens automatically. Reduced function becomes associated with reduced effort. Difficulty concentrating becomes associated with insufficient discipline. Physical heaviness becomes associated with laziness. The inability to sustain output across time becomes framed as weakness, low motivation, or lack of resilience. In many environments, fatigue is treated less as information from the body and more as evidence about character. The experience becomes personalized immediately.

This interpretation creates distortion because fatigue is not primarily a moral signal. It is not a behavioral verdict generated to evaluate worth, determination, intelligence, ambition, or value. Fatigue is a system signal. It reflects conditions inside the body that alter usable function, available capacity, recovery state, resource allocation, and output sustainability across time.

That distinction changes the entire framework through which fatigue is understood.

A system signal is not meaningless simply because it is subjective. Many important physiological signals are experienced before they are measured. Hunger, thirst, pain, dizziness, heaviness, alertness, temperature discomfort, and breathlessness all exist partly through experience. Fatigue belongs to this category. It is experiential, but experience does not make it imaginary. The fact that fatigue can be difficult to quantify does not remove its informational value.

The body continuously regulates energy availability, repair demand, stress adaptation, fuel allocation, sleep recovery, fluid balance, glucose distribution, and nervous system signaling. These systems interact constantly. Fatigue emerges partly from the interaction between demand and available capacity within those systems. When the relationship between load and capacity changes, the experience of usable function changes with it.

This does not mean fatigue has a single cause. One of the reasons fatigue becomes confusing is because it is non-specific. The same broad sensation may emerge from very different forms of strain. Inadequate recovery, prolonged stress exposure, sleep disruption, unstable glucose regulation, insufficient fuel availability, illness, inflammatory strain, psychological overload, electrolyte disruption, excessive demand, chronic under-recovery, and sustained compensatory effort can all alter system state in ways that produce fatigue signals.

Because fatigue is broad and non-specific, many people conclude that it is meaningless. The opposite is usually closer to reality. Broad signals often indicate system-wide integration rather than isolated malfunction. Fatigue is not useful because it identifies a precise mechanism instantly. It is useful because it indicates that capacity, recovery, or regulation may no longer be aligned with current demand.

A warning light on a dashboard does not explain the entire mechanical state of a vehicle, but it still communicates that interpretation is necessary. Fatigue functions similarly. The signal may require context before it becomes clear, but ambiguity does not eliminate significance.

Modern interpretations of fatigue often collapse into two extremes. One extreme dismisses fatigue entirely. The signal is ignored, overridden, minimized, or reframed as weakness. In this model, fatigue becomes an obstacle to productivity rather than information about system condition. Output is prioritized while interpretation disappears. The body's reduction in usable function is treated as something to suppress rather than understand.

The opposite extreme over-identifies with fatigue completely. Every fluctuation becomes catastrophic. Temporary reductions in capacity become interpreted as irreversible decline. Normal variability becomes medicalized immediately. Ordinary stress responses become signs of permanent dysfunction. In this model, fatigue stops being information and becomes identity.

Neither interpretation is stable because both remove context.

Ignoring fatigue disconnects output from capacity. Over-identifying with fatigue disconnects interpretation from proportionality. In both cases, the signal loses usefulness.

Fatigue becomes more interpretable when it is understood as part of a broader system state rather than as an isolated event. A single exhausted afternoon means less than a recurring pattern connected to poor sleep, prolonged stress exposure, unstable eating structure, sustained cognitive demand, illness recovery, or accumulated recovery debt. The signal gains meaning through continuity, interaction, timing, and persistence across time.

This is one reason fatigue often becomes more visible during periods of cumulative strain rather than during isolated high-demand moments. Acute stress can temporarily suppress fatigue signals through compensatory activation. Increased stress hormones, heightened alertness, urgency, novelty, or emotional intensity can temporarily maintain output despite rising strain. Function appears preserved even while recovery debt accumulates underneath.

Eventually the system loses the ability to compensate cleanly. Output becomes more difficult to sustain. Recovery becomes less complete. Variability increases. Cognitive clarity declines. Physical heaviness increases. Emotional tolerance narrows. Motivation becomes unstable. Small demands begin consuming disproportionate capacity. Fatigue becomes more visible not because the person suddenly became weaker, but because the gap between demand and recoverable function widened beyond what compensation could continue masking.

This distinction matters because people often misinterpret delayed fatigue as sudden failure. In reality, many forms of fatigue emerge gradually through accumulation.

Recovery debt is one of the clearest examples. Recovery is not a singular event accomplished fully each night. It is an ongoing restorative process distributed across sleep quality, nervous system downregulation, nutritional sufficiency, glucose stability, hormonal coordination, stress reduction, fluid balance, tissue repair, and overall load management. When recovery repeatedly fails to match demand, strain accumulates faster than restoration. Fatigue frequently reflects this imbalance long before complete functional breakdown occurs.

The body adapts remarkably well to temporary strain. Short periods of reduced sleep, increased workload, emotional stress, illness, travel, or elevated demand are often manageable because the system can absorb temporary instability. Problems emerge when temporary strain becomes persistent while recovery remains incomplete. The body then reallocates resources toward continuity rather than optimization. Available function narrows. Stability margins shrink. Fatigue signals increase because the system is attempting to regulate output relative to constrained capacity.

This makes fatigue protective in many contexts rather than obstructive. A reduction in available function is not always evidence that the body is malfunctioning irrationally. Sometimes the reduction represents adaptation under strain. When resources become constrained, the system may downshift output in order to preserve continuity elsewhere. Physical slowing, reduced motivation, increased heaviness, cognitive fog, lower tolerance for stimulation, and decreased voluntary activity can all function partly as energy conservation responses under conditions of accumulated strain.

That does not mean all fatigue should be normalized casually. Persistent, severe, unusual, rapidly worsening, or unexplained fatigue should not be dismissed and may require appropriate medical evaluation. The purpose of interpreting fatigue as a system signal is not to trivialize serious conditions. It is to prevent reflexive moralization while preserving careful interpretation.

Moral interpretations of fatigue create additional strain because they transform physiological limitation into personal accusation. Once fatigue becomes associated with failure, people often respond through escalation. More stimulants, more pressure, more suppression, more self-criticism, more forced output, more override behavior. Temporary increases in performance may occur, but the underlying strain frequently remains unresolved. The system is asked to produce greater output while already signaling reduced recoverable capacity.

Over time, this widens the mismatch between visible performance and underlying stability.

Many people become disconnected from fatigue gradually because continuous strain alters baseline expectations. Constant tiredness becomes normalized. Low-grade exhaustion becomes interpreted as adulthood, ambition, responsibility, or personal inadequacy rather than as information about sustained load. The signal remains present, but interpretation changes. Fatigue becomes background noise.

This normalization creates another problem: once exhaustion becomes habitual, people often stop recognizing variability altogether. They no longer compare current function to stable recovery states because stable recovery has become unfamiliar. The system adapts to chronic strain until reduced function feels ordinary.

In this environment, fatigue often becomes visible only when compensation fails dramatically. A person who has operated under sustained recovery debt for months or years may not notice gradual decline because the transition occurred incrementally. The eventual experience of collapse then appears sudden even though the underlying strain accumulated progressively across time.

The relationship between fatigue and fuel availability also complicates interpretation. Usable function depends partly on the ability to access and distribute energy efficiently relative to demand. Fatigue may emerge not only from insufficient intake, but also from unstable availability, impaired regulation, inconsistent timing, excessive variability, or difficulty transitioning between fuel states smoothly. When glucose regulation becomes unstable, for example, energy continuity often becomes less predictable. Rapid elevations and declines in glucose availability can alter perceived stability, concentration, mood, and physical function across time.

Similarly, electrolyte disruption can influence fatigue because electrical signaling depends on fluid and mineral balance across tissues. Muscle heaviness, nervous system slowing, reduced tolerance for activity, headaches, and generalized exhaustion may partly reflect impaired signal integrity rather than simple lack of effort. The experience still manifests as fatigue, but the underlying mechanism involves communication quality within the system rather than motivation failure.

Stress load also changes how fatigue appears. Stress is not purely psychological. It is physiological allocation. The body redistributes resources under perceived demand. Acute stress can temporarily increase available function, but persistent stress frequently increases baseline strain while reducing recovery efficiency. Sleep quality declines, glucose regulation becomes more volatile, nervous system activation remains elevated, and restorative processes become less complete. Fatigue then emerges not as isolated tiredness, but as cumulative strain distributed across multiple regulatory systems simultaneously.

This is why fatigue rarely behaves like a simple equation. The signal reflects interaction more than singularity.

Two people may experience similar levels of exhaustion with completely different underlying contributors. One may be under severe sleep disruption. Another may be carrying prolonged emotional stress. Another may be recovering from illness. Another may be operating under unstable fuel availability. Another may be functioning within persistent inflammatory or immune strain. Another may simply be sustaining demand far beyond recoverable capacity across time.

The body does not generate separate subjective categories for every mechanism involved. Instead, multiple strains often converge into overlapping experiences of reduced usable function.

This convergence frustrates people because modern culture prefers precision, immediate clarity, and direct causation. Fatigue resists all three. It is often gradual, layered, context-dependent, and interactive. Yet the absence of simplicity does not remove interpretive value.

The signal becomes more useful when the question changes from "What is wrong with me?" to "What might this state be communicating about strain, capacity, recovery, or system demand?"

That shift removes blame without removing seriousness.

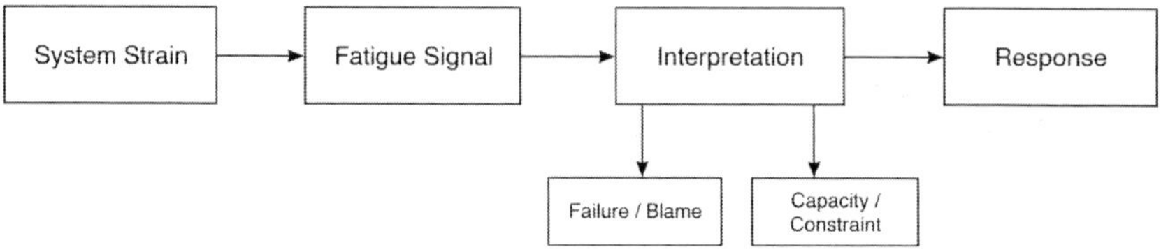


**[Figure 2: Fatigue Signal Pathway]**

The distinction represented here is small conceptually but enormous practically. Once fatigue passes through the interpretation layer, the response pattern changes dramatically. If fatigue is interpreted as personal failure, the response often becomes shame, suppression, escalation, or self-criticism. The signal generates conflict. The body communicates strain while the interpretation layer demands override.

If fatigue is interpreted as capacity and constraint information, the signal becomes contextual instead of moralized. Interpretation becomes observational rather than accusatory. The experience no longer needs to define identity in order to be taken seriously.

This does not mean every episode of fatigue requires intense analysis. Human function naturally fluctuates. Temporary tiredness after poor sleep, high demand, illness recovery, emotional strain, travel, or concentrated effort is part of normal physiology. Stable systems are not systems without fluctuation. They are systems capable of adapting and recovering without excessive breakdown.

The problem emerges when interpretation disconnects entirely from system reality. Persistent override behavior eventually increases strain because the body cannot indefinitely sustain output independent of recovery state. Likewise, catastrophic interpretation increases instability because fear amplifies monitoring, stress activation, and hypervigilance around ordinary fluctuations.

Fatigue becomes more manageable intellectually when it is removed from identity language. The experience may still be uncomfortable, disruptive, frustrating, or limiting, but it no longer automatically implies weakness or inadequacy. The signal can then be interpreted more clearly.

This reframing also restores proportionality. A person can acknowledge fatigue without collapsing into either dismissal or panic. The signal becomes part of understanding system condition rather than proof of failure.

Across time, this interpretive shift matters because fatigue influences behavior indirectly. Persistent strain alters decision-making, movement patterns, emotional regulation, attention, appetite, sleep behavior, and recovery capacity itself. When fatigue signals are repeatedly misread, compensatory patterns often develop around the misunderstanding. Increased stimulant reliance, irregular recovery behavior, unstable eating patterns, excessive suppression, emotional self-criticism, and oscillation between overexertion and collapse frequently emerge from the attempt to escape the signal without interpreting it.

The system then becomes progressively harder to read because compensation layers accumulate on top of original strain.

Understanding fatigue as information does not instantly resolve exhaustion. The signal is not eliminated merely because interpretation improves. But accurate interpretation changes the relationship between the person and the signal itself. Fatigue stops functioning as evidence of moral inadequacy and begins functioning as data about system state.

That distinction is foundational because fatigue is not merely about feeling tired. It is about the relationship between available capacity and current demand. The body continuously regulates output relative to recoverable function, resource availability, stress exposure, and stability margins across time. Fatigue becomes visible partly when those relationships narrow beyond what the system can sustain comfortably.

The signal therefore deserves neither shame nor dramatization. It deserves interpretation.

And once fatigue is understood as information rather than failure, a new question naturally emerges. If the system is reducing usable function, what kind of constraint is it attempting to communicate through that reduction?

# Output Constraint Mechanism

Fatigue is often interpreted as a failure of intention because intention is usually experienced more directly than capacity. A person decides to work, move, focus, respond, exercise, think clearly, remain patient, or continue performing across time. When the body does not fully cooperate with that intention, the experience feels personal. The gap between desired output and available function is interpreted as unwillingness, weakness, laziness, lack of motivation, or insufficient discipline because the internal desire to continue still exists while the usable ability to continue has narrowed.

This interpretation creates confusion because output is not generated through intention alone. Intention matters, but intention operates inside physiological conditions that determine whether sustained function can actually be supported. The body continuously regulates access to output relative to available resources, recovery state, stress burden, fuel accessibility, nervous system signaling quality, and overall support capacity. When those conditions deteriorate, available output often narrows even when desire remains intact.

This distinction becomes easier to recognize when observing fatigue directly. Many fatigued individuals do not lack intention. They often want very strongly to function normally. They want to think clearly, remain emotionally stable, complete ordinary responsibilities, maintain concentration, tolerate stimulation, and sustain physical movement without disproportionate effort. The frustration emerges precisely because intention remains present while usable function declines.

The mind interprets this conflict emotionally because modern culture often assumes output is voluntary in a near-absolute sense. Productivity models frequently imply that performance exists primarily as a consequence of mindset, discipline, or effort allocation. Within that framework, reduced output appears morally suspicious. If someone cannot sustain normal function, the assumption becomes that they are not trying hard enough or organizing themselves correctly.

Physiology does not operate according to that model.

The body regulates output continuously. Access to exertion, cognitive sharpness, emotional tolerance, speed, motivation, and sustained activity all depend on whether the system can support the energetic and regulatory cost required to maintain them. Output is permitted when conditions allow stable continuation. When support capacity narrows, output often narrows alongside it.

This narrowing is frequently experienced as fatigue.

The Output Constraint Mechanism describes this process directly: fatigue often appears when the body narrows access to usable function because current demand exceeds the support capacity required to sustain that output.

The important distinction inside this mechanism is that fatigue is not merely the presence of discomfort. It is often the reduction of accessible function itself. The system becomes less willing to allocate resources toward sustained output because the conditions necessary to support that output have become constrained.

This is why ordinary tasks can begin feeling disproportionately demanding under fatigue. The task itself may not have changed significantly. What changed is the relationship between demand and available support capacity. Activities that once existed comfortably within the system's tolerance range now consume a much larger percentage of available resources.

A conversation requires more effort. Concentration deteriorates more quickly. Physical movement feels heavier. Minor stressors become harder to absorb. Decision-making slows. Emotional regulation weakens. Cognitive endurance declines. Motivation becomes unstable not because character disappeared, but because motivation itself requires physiological support to remain accessible.

This creates one of the most misunderstood aspects of fatigue: the difference between unwillingness and constrained capacity.

Unwillingness refers primarily to the absence of desire or intention. Constrained capacity refers to the reduced ability to convert intention into sustained function. These states may appear superficially similar from the outside because both can produce reduced visible output. Internally, however, they are fundamentally different experiences.

A fatigued person often continues attempting to access normal function long after the system has begun narrowing available output. This creates friction between desired activity and supported activity. The individual experiences this friction as heaviness, effort amplification, slowing, irritability, reduced tolerance, mental fog, physical reluctance, or disproportionate exhaustion following ordinary demands.

The body is not necessarily refusing output irrationally. In many cases, it is regulating output relative to constrained support conditions.

Support capacity includes far more than immediate energy availability. The body's ability to sustain output depends on integrated recovery processes operating across multiple systems simultaneously. Sleep quality, nervous system regulation, glucose stability, fuel accessibility, stress burden, hydration status, electrolyte signaling integrity, hormonal coordination, immune activity, tissue repair demands, emotional strain, and prior exertion all influence how much output can be supported without destabilization.

When these layers remain relatively stable, the body can permit broader access to exertion and sustained function. When they become constrained, the system often downshifts.

This downshift is not always dramatic initially. Fatigue frequently develops through gradual narrowing rather than sudden collapse. Small reductions in available function accumulate across time. Focus becomes slightly harder to maintain. Recovery becomes less complete. Patience shortens. Motivation fluctuates more unpredictably. Cognitive flexibility decreases. Stress tolerance weakens. Physical movement feels less automatic.

Because these shifts often emerge progressively, people frequently adapt to declining function without recognizing the degree of accumulated strain involved. The system compensates temporarily. Output remains possible, but the regulatory cost rises steadily underneath.

Eventually the body begins protecting stability more aggressively by narrowing access to output itself.

This protective aspect of fatigue is important because many interpretations frame reduced function as punishment rather than regulation. The body is imagined as obstructing productivity, withholding energy unfairly, or failing to cooperate with conscious goals. In reality, reduced output often reflects an attempt to preserve continuity under constrained conditions.

Sustained output is metabolically expensive. Concentration requires regulatory coordination. Emotional stability requires nervous system flexibility. Physical exertion requires fuel access, fluid balance, neurological signaling, and recovery support. Even ordinary decision-making consumes physiological resources. The body continuously evaluates whether current conditions can support these demands without excessive destabilization.

When recoverable capacity narrows, unrestricted output may no longer be sustainable safely across time. The system then limits access to preserve broader stability.

This becomes especially visible under prolonged recovery debt. Recovery debt accumulates when restorative processes repeatedly fail to fully offset current demand. Sleep disruption, persistent stress activation, illness recovery, unstable nutrition, emotional overload, excessive exertion, and chronic under-recovery all contribute to this accumulation.

Importantly, recovery debt does not always feel dramatic initially. The body can compensate for temporary deficits remarkably well. Short-term sleep reduction, acute stress exposure, concentrated work periods, travel strain, or elevated cognitive demand may remain manageable for a while because compensatory systems temporarily preserve output.

Stress hormones increase alertness. Motivation intensifies temporarily. Urgency suppresses awareness of exhaustion. Adrenal activation increases short-term functionality despite rising strain underneath.

Eventually compensation becomes more difficult to sustain cleanly. The body then begins reducing accessible output because continuing at previous levels would require regulatory costs the system can no longer support comfortably.

The experience is often interpreted psychologically because the symptoms appear behavioral. A person cannot focus normally. They lose patience more quickly. They avoid effortful tasks. They move more slowly. They withdraw from stimulation. They procrastinate more frequently. They become emotionally reactive or mentally flat.

These changes are often treated as evidence of deteriorating character when they may instead represent deteriorating support conditions.

Fatigue frequently alters the perceived cost of action itself. Tasks that previously felt neutral begin carrying exaggerated effort signals. The brain and body increase resistance to exertion because exertion now consumes a larger proportion of available capacity. The individual experiences this as reluctance, heaviness, or inability to initiate. Externally, this can resemble low motivation. Internally, it often reflects constrained support capacity beneath the action.

This distinction matters because people commonly respond to fatigue by escalating pressure against themselves. More self-criticism, more forcing, more override behavior, more stimulatory compensation, more suppression of recovery signals. Temporary increases in output may occur, but the underlying mismatch between demand and support capacity often remains unresolved.

Over time, this strategy can widen instability because the body continues spending resources faster than recovery processes can restore them.

The relationship between sleep and output constraint illustrates this clearly. Sleep is not passive inactivity. It is active restoration. Neurological recovery, metabolic regulation, memory consolidation, hormonal coordination, immune modulation, tissue repair, and nervous system recalibration all depend heavily on sleep quality and continuity.

When sleep becomes fragmented, shortened, delayed, inconsistent, or physiologically poor, support capacity narrows even if conscious intention remains strong. A person may still want to perform normally, but the underlying system has reduced access to recoverable function. Cognitive endurance declines. Emotional tolerance narrows. Attention destabilizes. Physical fatigue rises. Stress reactivity increases. Recovery debt accumulates faster than restoration can offset it.

The resulting fatigue is not imaginary and not purely psychological. It is reduced accessible output under constrained restorative conditions.

Glucose instability can create similar effects through different pathways. Stable function depends partly on predictable fuel accessibility across time. When glucose regulation becomes highly volatile, usable function often becomes less continuous. Rapid elevations followed by steep declines may increase perceived crashes, cognitive inconsistency, irritability, shakiness, mental fog, or unstable energy continuity. The body then allocates resources under increasingly unpredictable conditions.

Fatigue emerges partly because stable output becomes more difficult to sustain when fuel access itself becomes unstable.

This does not mean fatigue is reducible to glucose alone. The mechanism is broader than any single variable. The body integrates multiple signals simultaneously when determining how much output can be safely supported.

Electrolyte signaling integrity also influences available function because cellular communication depends on stable electrical gradients and fluid distribution. Neuromuscular signaling, cardiac function, nerve transmission, and tissue coordination all require precise regulation. When signal quality deteriorates, output efficiency often declines. Heaviness, weakness, slowed function, headaches, mental dullness, and reduced exertional tolerance may emerge not because effort disappeared, but because signal transmission itself became less stable.

Stress load compounds these constraints further because chronic stress increases regulatory demand continuously. Persistent stress activation reallocates resources toward vigilance and adaptation. Sleep quality often deteriorates. Recovery efficiency declines. Glucose regulation becomes less stable. Muscular tension increases. Cognitive flexibility narrows. Emotional regulation becomes more effortful.

The body then attempts to maintain continuity while carrying elevated baseline load. Eventually output is narrowed because maintaining previous levels would exceed recoverable capacity.

This is one reason fatigue often feels disproportionate relative to visible activity. A person may appear physically inactive while still carrying enormous physiological load internally. Emotional strain, chronic uncertainty, persistent vigilance, illness recovery, inflammatory activation, disrupted sleep, cognitive overload, and ongoing stress adaptation all consume support capacity even without visible exertion.

The system responds to total load, not merely visible movement.

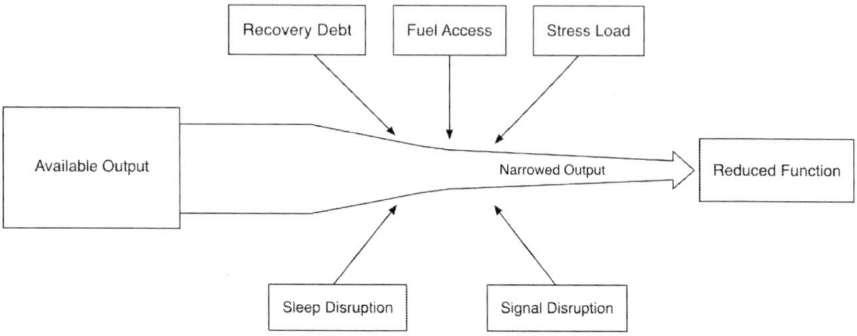


**[Figure 3: Output Constraint Model]**

The narrowing represented here is not conceptual abstraction alone. It reflects how fatigue frequently behaves experientially. Output begins broad when support capacity is relatively stable. As recovery debt, stress burden, fuel instability, sleep disruption, and signaling strain accumulate, available function narrows progressively. The resulting reduction in output is then experienced as fatigue, heaviness, slowed cognition, reduced tolerance, emotional fragility, or disproportionate effort cost.

The important implication is that reduced function may represent regulation rather than failure.

Constraint exists throughout physiology as a stability-preserving process. Pain limits movement under injury. Breathlessness limits exertion under respiratory strain. Hunger encourages energy intake under fuel need. Thirst encourages fluid restoration under hydration demand. Fatigue similarly appears partly as a mechanism that reduces access to output when continuing at current levels threatens broader stability.

This does not mean every fatigue signal is perfectly calibrated or always protective in an ideal sense. Human physiology is complex, adaptive, and sometimes imperfect. But broadly speaking, fatigue often emerges because the body is attempting to regulate exertion relative to recoverable support conditions.

The misunderstanding occurs because modern environments frequently separate output expectations from physiological realities. The body is expected to maintain continuous performance regardless of sleep quality, emotional load, recovery debt, illness recovery, cognitive demand, environmental stress, or metabolic instability. When output inevitably narrows under these conditions, the reduction is interpreted morally rather than physiologically.

This moralization increases confusion because shame obscures interpretation. Once fatigue becomes associated with inadequacy, individuals often stop examining the actual conditions shaping available function. The signal becomes personalized instead of contextualized.

The Output Constraint Mechanism restores context. Fatigue is not merely the feeling of wanting to rest. It is often the body narrowing access to usable function because current support conditions cannot sustain previous output safely across time.

That narrowing may appear cognitively through reduced focus and slower processing. It may appear emotionally through lower tolerance and increased reactivity. It may appear physically through heaviness, slowed movement, and reduced exertional endurance. It may appear behaviorally through avoidance of high-cost tasks because the physiological price of those tasks has risen relative to available capacity.

The visible behavior matters less than the underlying relationship between demand and support capacity producing it.

This distinction also explains why recovery sometimes restores function rapidly after prolonged exhaustion. The person did not suddenly acquire better character overnight. Support conditions improved enough for the body to widen access to output again. Sleep improved. Stress load declined. Illness resolved. Fuel access stabilized. Recovery debt decreased. Signal integrity improved. Capacity widened, and output followed.

The reverse occurs as well. A highly motivated person can become profoundly fatigued under sufficient strain because output is not determined by motivation alone. The body still regulates access according to recoverable support conditions.

Understanding fatigue through this lens changes interpretation fundamentally. Reduced output no longer automatically implies unwillingness. The question shifts away from accusation and toward regulation. What conditions are increasing total load? What conditions are narrowing support capacity? What forms of strain are elevating the regulatory cost of ordinary function?

These questions are more useful because they align fatigue with physiology instead of morality.

Fatigue is therefore not simply the absence of energy. It is often the narrowing of accessible function under constrained support conditions. The body reduces available output because sustaining previous levels would exceed what current recovery, regulation, and resource conditions can safely maintain across time.

The signal may feel frustrating, limiting, or disruptive, but it is not necessarily evidence of laziness or failure. It is frequently evidence that the system is attempting to preserve continuity under strain.

And once fatigue is understood as constrained output rather than unwillingness, another layer becomes visible underneath it. Output limitation does not occur randomly. The body regulates available function relative to the relationship between total load and remaining capacity.

# Load-Capacity Mismatch Mechanism

Fatigue is often treated as a singular sensation, but the experience becomes more understandable when viewed as a relationship rather than an isolated feeling. The body does not generate fatigue randomly or independently from conditions surrounding it. Fatigue emerges through interaction. Demand rises, capacity narrows, recovery becomes incomplete, regulation costs increase, and the relationship between what the system is carrying and what it can sustainably support begins to drift out of alignment.

This drift is frequently experienced before it is recognized intellectually. A person notices that ordinary responsibilities feel heavier than they once did. Small tasks require disproportionate effort. Concentration fades earlier. Emotional tolerance shortens. Recovery from routine demands takes longer. Rest feels less restorative. Motivation becomes inconsistent. The visible activities themselves may not appear extreme, yet the internal experience of carrying them changes substantially.

The change occurs because fatigue is not determined solely by the size of a task. It is determined partly by the relationship between the task and the condition of the system performing it.

A staircase climbed after restorative sleep, stable nutrition, emotional calm, adequate hydration, and reasonable recovery debt may feel almost effortless. The same staircase climbed under severe sleep disruption, prolonged stress exposure, illness recovery, unstable glucose regulation, emotional overload, and accumulated fatigue may feel disproportionately demanding. The staircase did not change. The system state carrying the staircase changed.

This distinction is central to understanding fatigue accurately because most interpretations focus too heavily on visible demand while overlooking available capacity. Human beings tend to evaluate effort externally. Tasks are judged according to what they appear to require objectively. If a demand seems small from the outside, fatigue in response to it is often interpreted as excessive or illegitimate.

Physiology does not evaluate demand that way.

The body responds to total load relative to available support capacity. A task exists inside a larger system state that includes sleep quality, recovery debt, emotional strain, fuel availability, nervous system regulation, metabolic stability, prior exertion, illness burden, environmental stress, and ongoing adaptation demands. The visible activity is only one portion of the total equation.

This is why fatigue can become confusing in modern environments. Many forms of load are invisible. Physical exertion is easy to recognize because it can be observed directly. Heavy lifting, prolonged activity, intense exercise, physical labor, and movement across time all visibly consume energy and resources. Mental, emotional, regulatory, and metabolic loads are more difficult to observe externally even though they can consume enormous capacity internally.

Cognitive demand alone can produce substantial fatigue under certain conditions. Sustained concentration requires continuous regulation. Attention must be maintained. Competing stimuli must be filtered. Decisions must be processed. Emotional responses must be moderated. Memory must remain accessible. Stress signals must be interpreted. Social interaction must be managed. The nervous system continuously allocates resources toward maintaining coherence across these processes.

Under stable conditions, much of this regulation occurs efficiently enough that the cost remains relatively invisible. Under strain, the cost becomes increasingly apparent. Concentration shortens. Decision fatigue rises. Small interruptions become disproportionately disruptive. Ordinary conversations feel effortful. Tolerance for complexity narrows. Cognitive output begins consuming more of the available system capacity.

Emotional load functions similarly. Emotional strain is not merely a psychological abstraction. Persistent uncertainty, vigilance, grief, conflict, pressure, instability, anticipation, suppression, or unresolved stress all increase regulatory demand across time. The body does not separate emotional experience from physiology cleanly. Stress responses alter hormonal signaling, sleep quality, muscular tension, nervous system activation, glucose regulation, inflammatory activity, and recovery efficiency.

A person carrying prolonged emotional strain may therefore experience fatigue even in the absence of substantial physical exertion because the system is already operating under elevated baseline demand.

Metabolic load also contributes heavily to fatigue while often remaining misunderstood. The body must continuously regulate fuel availability, glucose distribution, tissue energy access, fluid balance, electrolyte signaling, digestion, repair processes, temperature regulation, immune activity, and countless other background functions required for stability. These processes consume regulatory resources continuously even when they are not consciously noticed.

When glucose becomes highly unstable, for example, the body may spend increasing effort attempting to stabilize fuel availability across time. Rapid elevations and declines in available glucose can increase perceived instability, disrupt continuity of usable energy, and raise overall regulation cost. Similarly, disrupted fluid balance or impaired electrolyte signaling can reduce the efficiency of communication across tissues, increasing the effort required to maintain stable function.

The body therefore carries both visible and invisible forms of demand simultaneously.

This becomes important because people often underestimate total system load by focusing only on externally measurable activity. A person may believe they "did very little" during a day while the body experienced enormous cumulative strain internally through poor sleep, prolonged stress activation, emotional overload, unstable fuel regulation, illness recovery, inflammatory burden, and continuous nervous system vigilance.

The body responds to total strain, not merely visible movement.

The Load-Capacity Mismatch Mechanism describes this relationship directly: fatigue appears when total demand exceeds or approaches the available capacity required to sustain output without excessive destabilization.

The word "approaches" matters almost as much as the word "exceeds." Fatigue often becomes visible before total collapse occurs. Systems do not usually move instantly from stability into complete breakdown. More often, the stability margin gradually narrows. Ordinary demands begin consuming a larger proportion of available capacity. Recovery becomes less complete. Variability increases. The cost of maintaining ordinary function rises steadily beneath the surface.

Eventually the mismatch becomes difficult to ignore because the system no longer possesses enough reserve capacity to absorb ordinary fluctuation comfortably.

This explains why fatigue frequently appears gradual in retrospect even when it feels sudden in the moment. The mismatch often develops progressively through accumulation. Sleep quality deteriorates slowly. Stress load persists longer than expected. Recovery periods become shorter or less effective. Fuel instability becomes more frequent. Emotional strain remains unresolved. Workload increases incrementally. Illness recovery remains incomplete. The nervous system remains activated for prolonged periods.

At first, compensation preserves function relatively well. The body adapts temporarily. Increased stress activation can maintain alertness.

Urgency can suppress awareness of exhaustion. Motivation can temporarily override strain signals. Short-term compensation allows output to continue even while underlying capacity narrows.

Eventually compensation itself becomes expensive. The body begins reducing accessible output because maintaining prior levels now requires regulatory costs that exceed recoverable support conditions. Fatigue then emerges more visibly not because the person suddenly became weaker, but because the mismatch between load and capacity widened beyond what compensation could continue masking.

This is one reason highly capable or highly motivated individuals can experience profound fatigue. Strong intention does not eliminate physiological mismatch. In some cases, high motivation can temporarily conceal mismatch longer by increasing override behavior and suppressing awareness of accumulating strain. The eventual fatigue may then appear disproportionate or confusing because the visible collapse seems disconnected from earlier functioning.

In reality, the mismatch had often been developing gradually beneath the preserved performance.

Capacity itself is dynamic rather than fixed. The body does not maintain identical support capacity across all conditions and all periods of life. Capacity expands and contracts continuously depending on recovery state, sleep quality, fuel accessibility, stress exposure, emotional burden, prior exertion, adaptation history, illness status, hydration, electrolyte balance, environmental conditions, and overall system stability.

This variability explains why the same person can tolerate a demand comfortably in one condition and struggle severely with it in another. Capacity changed even if the visible task remained identical.

Sleep plays a particularly important role because restorative function depends heavily on sleep continuity and quality. Sleep is not passive absence of activity. It is active recalibration and recovery. Memory consolidation, tissue repair, hormonal coordination, immune regulation, nervous system downshifting, metabolic restoration, and emotional processing all depend heavily on adequate sleep architecture.

When sleep quality deteriorates, capacity narrows even if outward effort remains unchanged. The person may continue attempting to sustain normal demands, but ordinary activities now consume more of the reduced reserve available to support them. Fatigue emerges because demand and recoverable capacity are no longer aligned cleanly.

Recovery debt compounds this narrowing further. Recovery debt accumulates when restorative processes repeatedly fail to fully offset ongoing load. The system then begins each successive day carrying unresolved strain from prior demands. Capacity becomes progressively less available because restoration never fully catches up to expenditure.

This accumulation is often difficult to recognize initially because human beings adapt remarkably well to moderate instability. The body preserves continuity wherever possible. Function remains partially accessible. Responsibilities continue. Daily life proceeds outwardly.

Internally, however, the cost of maintaining that continuity may rise steadily.

Eventually ordinary demands begin feeling excessive because the available stability margin has narrowed too far. The mismatch becomes experiential. The individual feels fatigue not as abstract theory but as lived reduction in usable function.

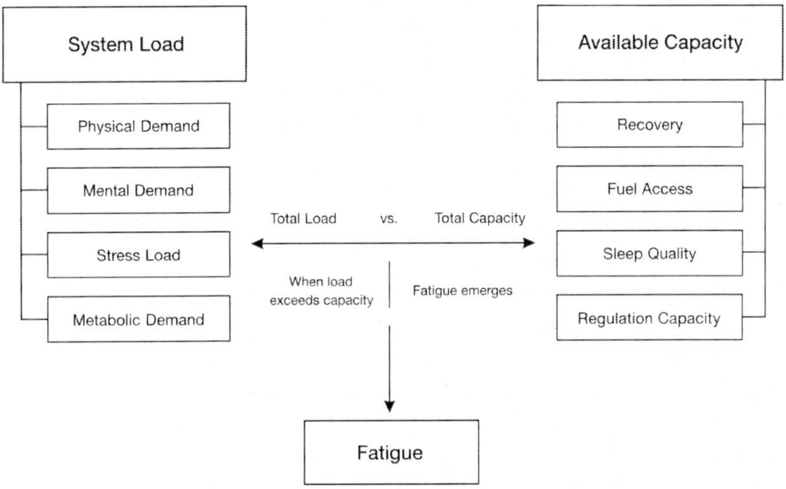


**[Figure 4: Load-Capacity Mismatch]**

The relationship represented here explains why fatigue cannot be understood accurately through visible effort alone. System load includes physical exertion, but it also includes mental demand, stress activation, emotional strain, metabolic regulation, and the background costs required to maintain stable function. Capacity depends on recovery, sleep quality, fuel access, regulation efficiency, nervous system stability, and the absence or presence of accumulated strain. When the load side widens while the capacity side narrows, fatigue emerges as the felt experience of mismatch.

Importantly, stable systems are not systems without demand. Stability does not require the elimination of effort, stress, challenge, exertion, complexity, or adaptation. Human physiology is designed to handle fluctuation, activity, and periods of elevated demand. Problems emerge primarily when demand remains persistently misaligned with the system's ability to recover and regulate effectively across time.

A stable system can tolerate substantial challenge because capacity remains sufficient relative to load. An unstable system may struggle under comparatively modest demands because the available margin has already narrowed.

This distinction removes moral interpretation from fatigue because it reframes exhaustion as relational rather than character-based. The question becomes less about toughness and more about alignment. How much total load is the system carrying? How much recoverable capacity remains available? How much reserve exists between current demand and destabilization?

These questions matter because increasing effort against constrained capacity often worsens mismatch rather than resolving it.

When fatigue is interpreted as weakness, people frequently respond through escalation. More pressure, more forcing, more override behavior, more suppression of exhaustion signals, more reliance on stimulatory compensation. Short-term output may increase temporarily, but the underlying relationship between load and capacity often deteriorates further because the body is spending resources faster than recovery processes can replenish them.

The mismatch widens silently underneath the preserved performance.

This pattern becomes especially dangerous when visible functioning remains relatively intact despite rising strain. Many people assume that continued output proves adequate capacity. Physiology does not necessarily operate that way. Compensation can preserve visible function for extended periods even while recovery debt accumulates steadily beneath the surface.

The eventual fatigue then appears disproportionate because the visible workload alone seems insufficient to explain the collapse. In reality, the body had often been operating near capacity limits for far longer than the person recognized consciously.

The nervous system plays a major role in this process because sustained vigilance and prolonged activation increase baseline regulation costs continuously. A system carrying chronic uncertainty, pressure, emotional tension, overstimulation, or unresolved stress remains partially activated even during periods that appear externally calm. Recovery becomes less complete because downshifting itself becomes more difficult.

The body then spends more energy maintaining readiness and less energy restoring stability. Capacity gradually narrows while baseline load remains elevated.

Adaptation complicates the picture further because human beings normalize strain remarkably quickly. Reduced function often becomes familiar before it becomes alarming. A person adjusts to persistent fatigue incrementally. Slightly lower concentration becomes normal. Slightly poorer recovery becomes expected. Slightly elevated irritability becomes ordinary. The baseline shifts quietly.

This normalization obscures mismatch because the person stops comparing current function against truly recovered conditions. The system adapts behaviorally even while carrying significant unresolved strain physiologically.

Fatigue then becomes visible primarily when the mismatch grows large enough that ordinary compensation no longer works effectively.

Understanding fatigue through the Load-Capacity Mismatch Mechanism changes interpretation fundamentally because the focus shifts away from isolated sensations and toward relationships inside the system. Fatigue is no longer viewed as a mysterious failure of motivation or character. It becomes the felt signal that total demand is approaching or exceeding what current recovery, regulation, and support conditions can sustain comfortably across time.

The signal may appear physically through heaviness and reduced exertional tolerance. It may appear cognitively through slowed concentration and reduced clarity. It may appear emotionally through shortened patience and lower resilience. It may appear behaviorally through increasing difficulty initiating or sustaining ordinary tasks.

The specific form matters less than the underlying mismatch producing it.

This interpretation also explains why relief sometimes occurs rapidly when capacity improves or load decreases. Sleep restores part of the reserve. Emotional strain eases. Illness resolves. Fuel stability improves. Recovery debt decreases. Nervous system activation downshifts. Capacity widens again, and ordinary demands consume a smaller proportion of available support.

The person does not suddenly become morally stronger. The relationship between load and capacity changes.

Fatigue therefore deserves contextual interpretation rather than blame. The body is not simply reporting effort. It is reporting the relationship between total demand and available support conditions required to sustain that demand without excessive destabilization.

And once fatigue is understood as the felt experience of mismatch, another important question emerges naturally underneath it. Capacity depends not only on recovery and regulation, but also on whether usable fuel can actually be accessed reliably when needed. Stored energy alone does not guarantee stable usable energy.

## Fuel Availability Mechanism

Fatigue is often described as low energy, but the phrase becomes misleading when energy is treated only as quantity. The human body can contain substantial stored energy while still experiencing periods of unstable or insufficient usable function. This apparent contradiction confuses many interpretations of fatigue because the visible existence of stored fuel is assumed to guarantee continuous access to usable energy. Physiology operates more dynamically than that.

Stored energy and available energy are not identical conditions.

The body continuously stores, releases, transports, regulates, distributes, and allocates fuel across changing states of demand. Energy must not only exist somewhere within the system. It must also become accessible at the appropriate time, in the appropriate form, at the appropriate rate, and in coordination with the demands currently being placed on the body. Fatigue can therefore emerge not only from absolute deficiency, but from inconsistency, delay, instability, or mismatch in usable fuel access.

This distinction matters because many experiences of fatigue occur in situations where fuel technically exists within the body. Glycogen may be present. Fat stores may be substantial. Recent intake may have occurred. Yet concentration deteriorates, heaviness develops, output becomes unstable, irritability rises, and ordinary activity begins feeling disproportionately demanding.

The problem in these situations is often less about the total existence of energy and more about the regulation of availability.

The Fuel Availability Mechanism describes this directly: fatigue can appear when usable fuel is not consistently accessible at the time, intensity, or location where function requires it.

This mechanism shifts the interpretation of fatigue away from simplistic ideas of energy absence. The body is not a static reservoir where stored calories automatically translate into continuous usable function. Fuel access depends on coordinated regulation involving feeding state, fasting state, glucose stability, insulin signaling, liver glucose release, nervous system activity, metabolic flexibility, stress load, and current demand.

The body must constantly match fuel availability to changing conditions. This matching process is dynamic because human demand is dynamic. Physical activity changes. Cognitive demand changes. Emotional strain changes. Stress exposure changes. Sleep quality changes. Recovery state changes. The body therefore continuously adjusts how fuel is stored, released, distributed, and utilized across time.

Under stable conditions, much of this process remains relatively invisible. Fuel arrives where it is needed with enough continuity that ordinary function feels smooth and sustainable. Concentration remains accessible. Physical movement feels proportionate to the task. Mood remains relatively stable. Energy continuity persists across changing demands.

When fuel access becomes inconsistent or poorly coordinated, the experience of function often changes before the underlying mechanism becomes obvious.

A person may feel mentally foggy despite adequate intake. Physical heaviness may emerge unexpectedly during ordinary activity. Irritability increases. Tolerance narrows. Energy becomes unstable across the day. Motivation fluctuates sharply. Output becomes difficult to sustain consistently. Fatigue appears not necessarily because the body lacks total energy, but because usable fuel availability has become unstable relative to demand.

This instability can emerge through several pathways simultaneously.

The feeding state and fasting state both influence how fuel becomes available. During feeding, incoming nutrients increase circulating fuel availability while insulin signaling helps coordinate storage, uptake, and distribution. During fasting, the body shifts toward maintaining fuel continuity through stored energy mobilization, liver glucose release, fatty acid utilization, and broader adaptive coordination.

Neither state is inherently problematic. Human physiology is designed to transition between them continuously. Fatigue often emerges not because either state exists, but because transitions between states become poorly coordinated relative to demand.

The body must maintain continuity during these transitions. Glucose availability must remain sufficiently stable. Liver release must remain responsive. Fat utilization must remain accessible when appropriate. Nervous system signaling must remain coordinated. Output demands must remain supportable relative to current fuel accessibility.

When this coordination becomes unstable, fatigue frequently becomes more visible.

One reason this instability becomes confusing is because stored energy can create the illusion that fuel access should always remain effortless. The body may possess substantial stored fat while still struggling to provide rapid usable energy under certain conditions. Fat storage and fat accessibility are not interchangeable. Stored fuel must still be mobilized, transported, regulated, and integrated into current energetic demands.

Similarly, recent intake does not guarantee stable usable function. Energy entering the body and energy becoming usable across tissues are related but distinct processes. Digestion, absorption, insulin signaling, glucose regulation, liver coordination, nervous system state, and current activity demand all influence how smoothly incoming fuel becomes available for sustained function.

This distinction becomes especially important during changing activity levels. The body constantly adjusts fuel utilization according to intensity, duration, and type of demand. Low-intensity activity, concentrated mental work, high-intensity exertion, emotional stress, and recovery states all influence how fuel is allocated and prioritized.

Under stable conditions, these adjustments occur with relatively little disruption. Under unstable conditions, the transitions themselves may become energetically expensive.

Metabolic flexibility plays a major role here because the body's ability to shift between fuel sources influences how smoothly energy continuity is maintained. Metabolic flexibility refers partly to the capacity to transition between glucose use, fat use, feeding states, fasting states, rest conditions, and activity demand without excessive disruption or instability.

When this flexibility narrows, fuel transitions often become less efficient. The body may struggle to shift cleanly between stored and incoming fuel sources. Delays emerge. Instability increases. Energy continuity becomes less reliable. Fatigue may then appear during periods when the system is attempting to transition between energetic states but cannot do so smoothly.

This experience is often interpreted incorrectly because people assume that if energy exists somewhere in the body, stable function should remain automatic. Physiologically, however, fuel must remain accessible in real time relative to changing demands.

A useful distinction exists between storage and flow. Stored fuel represents potential energy reserve. Usable fuel availability represents the active movement of energy through functioning systems. Fatigue often reflects disruptions in flow more than absolute absence of reserve.

The liver plays an especially important role in this continuity because it helps maintain glucose availability between feeding periods. Liver glucose release contributes to stable fuel accessibility during fasting states, overnight periods, and gaps between intake. This process helps preserve continuity when incoming fuel is temporarily absent.

When glucose regulation becomes unstable, however, the balance between incoming fuel, stored glycogen, liver release, insulin signaling, and tissue uptake may become more difficult to coordinate smoothly. The resulting instability can create fluctuations in concentration, irritability, heaviness, shakiness, reduced tolerance, and perceived energy continuity.

Importantly, this does not mean fatigue should be reduced simplistically to glucose alone. Fuel regulation is one layer inside a broader system involving recovery, stress adaptation, nervous system regulation, hormonal coordination, and overall support capacity. The Fuel Availability Mechanism explains one pathway through which fatigue may emerge, not the entirety of fatigue itself.

Stress load strongly influences this pathway because stress alters fuel regulation continuously. Acute stress can temporarily increase fuel mobilization and alertness in order to support immediate demand. Persistent stress exposure, however, often destabilizes fuel continuity across time. Sleep quality deteriorates. Nervous system activation remains elevated. Glucose variability increases. Recovery efficiency declines. The body spends more time managing vigilance and less time maintaining stable restoration.

Under these conditions, usable fuel availability may become increasingly inconsistent relative to ongoing demand.

Poor sleep compounds this instability further because sleep disruption alters both regulation quality and energetic continuity. Sleep loss changes glucose handling, stress signaling, recovery efficiency, appetite regulation, and nervous system stability simultaneously. The result is often increased variability in energy continuity rather than simple tiredness alone.

A person may therefore feel both fatigued and overstimulated simultaneously. Exhaustion coexists with restlessness. Cognitive slowing coexists with elevated stress activation. Energy feels unstable rather than absent. The system struggles to maintain coordinated fuel access across changing demands.

Recovery debt magnifies these effects because unresolved strain increases the cost of maintaining ordinary function. The body begins operating with narrower reserves while simultaneously requiring more regulation to preserve stability. Fuel demand rises while fuel coordination becomes less efficient. Fatigue then emerges partly because the energetic cost of maintaining continuity increases beyond what current regulation can support smoothly.

This is one reason ordinary tasks can suddenly feel disproportionately demanding under accumulated strain. The visible activity may appear unchanged, but the energetic cost of sustaining it has risen internally. More regulatory effort is required to maintain concentration, emotional stability, physical movement, and cognitive continuity. Fuel access becomes less predictable. Output becomes less stable.

The resulting fatigue often feels confusing because it does not resemble simple depletion. A person may experience fluctuating periods of temporary energy followed by rapid collapse. Brief alertness may alternate with heaviness and fog. Output may feel accessible temporarily and then disappear unexpectedly.

These fluctuations frequently reflect instability in usable fuel coordination rather than total absence of stored energy.

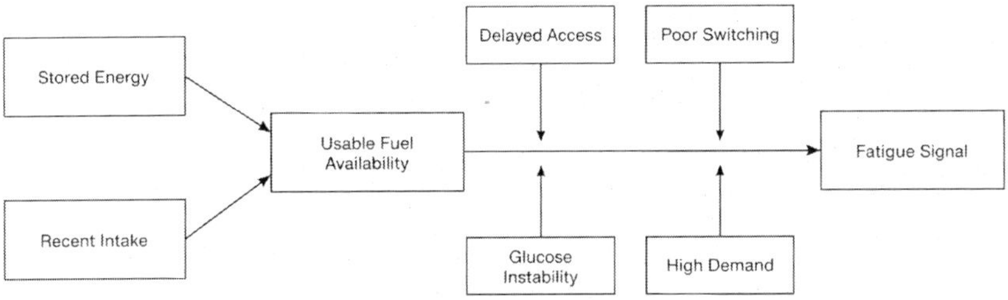


**[Figure 5: Fuel Availability Constraint]**

The relationship represented here clarifies why fatigue cannot be interpreted solely through the presence or absence of stored energy. Stored fuel and recent intake both contribute to usable fuel availability, but several constraints can interfere with smooth access. Delayed access, poor switching between fuel states, glucose instability, and rising demand can all narrow the continuity of usable energy delivery. Fatigue then emerges as the experiential signal of unstable access rather than absolute emptiness.

This distinction also explains why the same intake pattern or energetic condition may produce different experiences under different system states. A well-rested system with stable nervous system regulation, lower stress burden, and preserved metabolic flexibility may maintain smooth fuel continuity under conditions that would produce pronounced fatigue in a system carrying heavy recovery debt and elevated regulatory strain.

The context surrounding fuel matters as much as fuel itself.

This is why simplistic interpretations of fatigue through singular dietary rules often fail to explain lived experience accurately. Fatigue cannot be reduced cleanly to "eat more," "eat less," "avoid carbohydrates," "increase carbohydrates," "fast longer," "eat more frequently," or any other isolated lever. Human energy regulation operates through coordination rather than through a single variable.

Fuel availability depends on timing, regulation, distribution, nervous system state, hormonal signaling, metabolic flexibility, current demand, prior strain, and overall system stability. The same nutritional pattern may interact very differently with different physiological states because the system carrying the fuel is not identical in every condition.

The body therefore cannot be understood as a simple caloric machine. Energy accessibility is conditional. Stored energy must become usable energy within dynamic regulatory environments that are continuously adjusting to changing demands.

Fatigue emerges partly when those adjustments become unstable.

This instability becomes especially visible during transitions. Transitions between feeding and fasting states. Transitions between rest and activity. Transitions between low demand and high demand. Transitions between stress activation and recovery. The body must continually redistribute resources across these shifting conditions while preserving continuity.

When transitions remain smooth, fatigue remains less visible. When transitions become delayed, unstable, or poorly coordinated, fatigue often appears as heaviness, irritability, unstable output, mental fog, reduced tolerance, and disproportionate effort cost.

Importantly, the body is not malfunctioning merely because fatigue appears during these conditions. Fatigue frequently functions as information about current accessibility limits. The system is signaling that fuel continuity, regulation, or transition efficiency may no longer fully match present demand.

This interpretation matters because it removes moral framing from unstable energy experiences. A person experiencing inconsistent usable energy is not necessarily weak, lazy, undisciplined, or insufficiently motivated. The body may simply be operating under conditions where fuel access has become less coordinated relative to current demands.

Understanding this mechanism also clarifies why temporary stimulation often fails to resolve deeper fatigue cleanly. Alertness can sometimes be increased artificially even while underlying fuel instability remains unresolved. The person may feel temporarily more activated while still lacking smooth continuity of usable function. The resulting pattern often becomes one of oscillation rather than stability.

The deeper issue is not merely stimulation. It is coordinated accessibility.

The Fuel Availability Mechanism therefore reframes fatigue as an issue of timing, regulation, access, and distribution rather than simple absence of stored energy. Fatigue may emerge because usable fuel becomes inconsistent, delayed, poorly coordinated, or mismatched to the demands currently being placed on the system.

This does not make fuel availability the sole explanation for fatigue. Human exhaustion remains multi-layered, interactive, and context-dependent. Recovery debt, stress burden, nervous system strain, sleep disruption, illness, emotional overload, and broader capacity constraints all remain deeply relevant. Fuel accessibility is one mechanism inside a larger system.

But it is an important mechanism because the body cannot sustain stable output without stable access to usable energy across changing conditions.

And once fuel availability is understood as a problem of coordinated access rather than simple quantity, another layer becomes visible underneath fatigue itself. Even when usable fuel remains available, the physiological cost of producing stable function can rise dramatically under accumulated strain.

# Utilization Cost Mechanism

Fatigue is often interpreted through the question of whether enough energy exists, but the body does not operate only according to supply. Human function depends not merely on the presence of fuel, but on the ability to convert available resources into stable usable output efficiently across changing conditions. Energy production has operating costs. The body must coordinate fuel access, oxygen delivery, signaling integrity, nervous system regulation, fluid balance, tissue maintenance, immune activity, recovery processes, and stress adaptation continuously in order to sustain ordinary function.

Under stable conditions, much of this coordination remains relatively invisible. Function feels smooth enough that people rarely think about the regulatory expense required to produce it. Attention remains available. Physical movement feels proportionate to the task. Emotional tolerance remains reasonably stable. Cognitive effort does not feel excessively heavy. The body appears to generate usable function without obvious friction.

Under strain, this relationship changes. The system may still possess fuel availability while simultaneously requiring substantially greater effort to convert that fuel into stable function. Fatigue then emerges not necessarily because energy is absent, but because the operating cost of maintaining ordinary function has risen.

The Utilization Cost Mechanism describes this directly: fatigue can appear when the operating cost of producing usable function rises, reducing the amount of net function available from the same or similar fuel input.

This distinction matters because it explains forms of fatigue that feel heavy, inefficient, or disproportionately effortful even when fuel access appears relatively intact. A person may eat adequately, possess stored energy, and remain technically capable of performing tasks while still experiencing profound exhaustion. The experience often reflects rising regulatory expense rather than simple absence of energy supply.

Gross energy production and net usable function are not identical conditions.

The body continuously spends resources simply maintaining baseline stability. Heart rhythm must remain coordinated. Breathing must continue. Temperature must be regulated. Fluid distribution must remain balanced. Glucose must remain sufficiently stable. Muscles must maintain tone. Immune surveillance continues. Tissue repair occurs continuously. Nervous system signaling must remain coordinated. Hormonal communication must remain responsive.

All of these processes require energy expenditure before additional discretionary output such as concentration, emotional regulation, physical exertion, or complex decision-making even enters the picture.

Under stable conditions, the operating cost of maintaining these processes remains manageable relative to available support capacity. Under strain, the cost often rises substantially.

Stress load increases this expense quickly because stress is metabolically expensive. Acute stress temporarily reallocates resources toward vigilance, readiness, and rapid adaptation. This can preserve short-term function effectively under immediate demand. Persistent stress exposure, however, changes baseline regulation itself. Nervous system activation remains elevated. Sleep quality deteriorates. Muscular tension increases. Recovery efficiency declines. Glucose stability becomes more difficult to maintain.

Emotional regulation consumes more effort. Attention becomes more fragmented.

The body then spends increasing amounts of energy maintaining adaptation itself.

This distinction is important because visible output alone often fails to reveal how expensive that output has become internally. Two people may appear to complete the same task outwardly while carrying dramatically different utilization costs underneath. One system may perform the task smoothly with substantial reserve remaining. Another may complete the same activity while consuming most of its available stability margin in the process.

The visible action may look identical. The physiological cost is not.

This helps explain why fatigued individuals often describe ordinary activities as disproportionately draining. The activity itself may not be objectively extreme. What changed is the energetic expense required to sustain it. More regulation, more compensation, more effort, and more internal coordination are required simply to maintain ordinary continuity.

The body therefore feels inefficient not because it stopped producing energy entirely, but because increasing amounts of available resources are being redirected toward maintaining baseline stability under strain.

Poor sleep magnifies this effect significantly. Sleep is not simply passive rest. It is active restoration involving nervous system recalibration, hormonal coordination, glucose regulation, tissue repair, immune modulation, memory consolidation, and broader recovery processes. When sleep becomes fragmented, shortened, delayed, or physiologically poor, the body begins the following day carrying unresolved regulatory cost from the previous one.

This unresolved cost accumulates quietly. Concentration requires more effort. Emotional tolerance narrows more quickly. Physical exertion feels heavier. Cognitive flexibility declines. Stress sensitivity increases. The body spends greater energy maintaining ordinary function because restorative processes failed to fully reset the system.

The resulting fatigue often feels less like complete depletion and more like friction. Everything remains technically possible, but nothing feels metabolically inexpensive anymore.

Immune strain creates similar patterns through different pathways. The immune system requires substantial energetic support when activated. Illness recovery, chronic immune activation, unresolved inflammatory signaling, and ongoing repair processes all consume resources continuously. The body reallocates energy toward maintenance, defense, and restoration while simultaneously attempting to preserve ordinary function.

Fatigue then emerges partly because less net usable function remains available after these background regulatory costs are paid.

This experience is common during and after illness. Physical heaviness increases. Cognitive clarity declines. Emotional resilience narrows. Ordinary exertion becomes disproportionately tiring. The body may still contain adequate stored fuel, but a larger percentage of available resources is being consumed internally by regulation and recovery demands.

The same principle applies to prolonged recovery debt. Recovery debt is not merely the accumulation of tired feelings. It represents unresolved restorative cost carried forward across time. When recovery repeatedly fails to match ongoing demand, the body begins operating under elevated baseline strain continuously.

Under these conditions, maintaining ordinary function becomes progressively more expensive.

This rising cost explains why people often feel worse over time even while maintaining similar visible routines. The visible workload may appear stable, but the internal expense of sustaining that workload rises steadily underneath. More compensation is required. More regulation is required. More stress adaptation is required. More effort is required simply to preserve continuity.

Eventually the body begins reducing accessible output because the regulatory expense has become unsustainable relative to available support capacity.

This reduction frequently appears as fatigue long before total functional collapse occurs.

Glucose instability contributes to this process because unstable fuel regulation increases the cost of maintaining continuity. Rapid fluctuations in available fuel require additional corrective regulation. Stress signaling may increase. Nervous system activation may rise. Cognitive continuity may become less stable. Energy transitions become less smooth. The body spends more effort preserving basic stability across fluctuating conditions.

Fluid and electrolyte disruption can raise utilization cost similarly because signaling efficiency depends on stable electrical gradients and coordinated fluid distribution. Muscle contraction, nerve transmission, and broader tissue communication all depend on these relationships functioning efficiently. When signaling quality deteriorates, more effort may be required to produce the same visible output.

The resulting fatigue often feels heavy and resistant to simple stimulation because the issue is not merely alertness. The issue is rising operational expense underneath ordinary function.

This distinction helps explain why temporary stimulation frequently fails to resolve deeper exhaustion cleanly. Increased activation can temporarily increase alertness, urgency, or short-term output without actually lowering the cost of maintaining function. A person may feel temporarily more energized while still carrying elevated regulatory burden underneath.

The body therefore remains strained even when momentary activation masks the fatigue signal temporarily.

This pattern often creates oscillation. Temporary stimulation increases short-term output, but the underlying operating expense remains elevated. Recovery remains incomplete. Stress signaling remains high. Sleep quality often deteriorates further. The regulatory cost then accumulates even more aggressively afterward.

The issue is not merely how much energy enters the system. It is how much usable function remains available after regulatory costs are subtracted.

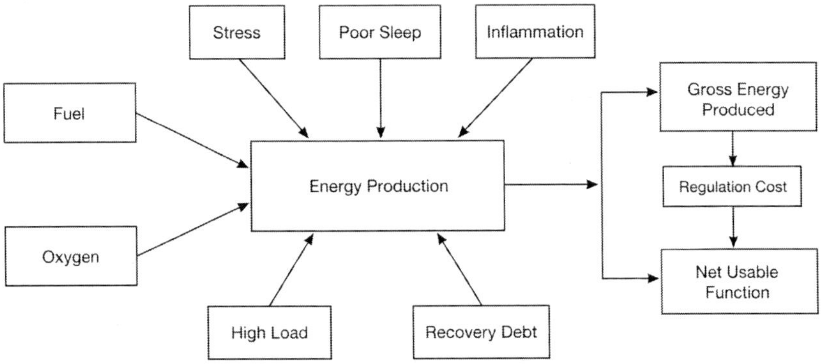


**[Figure 6: Utilization Cost Model]**

The relationship represented here clarifies why fatigue cannot be understood solely through fuel presence alone. Fuel and oxygen support energy production, but multiple conditions increase the regulatory expense required to turn that production into stable usable function. Stress load, poor sleep, immune strain, high ongoing demand, and accumulated recovery debt all raise operating cost. The body may continue producing gross energy while simultaneously delivering less net usable function because so many resources are being redirected toward maintaining stability itself.

This distinction becomes especially important when considering why fatigue can feel so disproportionate relative to visible activity. A person may appear inactive externally while internally carrying enormous regulatory expense. Persistent stress activation, immune recovery, poor sleep, emotional strain, unstable glucose regulation, and nervous system overload all consume energetic resources continuously even in the absence of obvious exertion.

The body therefore evaluates total operating burden rather than visible movement alone.

This is one reason people often become confused by exhaustion during periods that appear outwardly "less busy." The visible workload may have decreased while the invisible regulatory burden remained elevated or even increased. Recovery may still be incomplete. Stress signaling may still be active. Immune strain may still be present. Sleep quality may still be poor. The cost of producing stable function therefore remains high despite reduced visible activity.

The body responds to total regulatory demand, not merely external productivity.

Importantly, the Utilization Cost Mechanism should not become a singular explanation for all fatigue. Human exhaustion remains multi-layered and interactive. Fuel availability, recovery debt, emotional strain, sleep disruption, nervous system activation, illness burden, and broader load-capacity mismatch all interact continuously. Utilization cost explains one important layer: why the body may feel inefficient and disproportionately effortful even when fuel exists.

This mechanism also clarifies why fatigue often feels qualitatively different under different forms of strain. Some fatigue feels empty and depleted. Some feels unstable and inconsistent. Some feels heavy, dense, resistant, and metabolically expensive. The latter often reflects rising operating cost beneath ordinary function.

The body spends increasing amounts of available energy simply preserving continuity.

This preservation process is not irrational. Under strain, stability itself becomes more expensive to maintain. The body must regulate stress responses, preserve tissue integrity, maintain glucose continuity, support immune processes, coordinate signaling, stabilize fluid balance, and sustain basic cognitive coherence simultaneously. These processes consume resources before discretionary output is even considered.

The resulting fatigue therefore reflects reduced net usable function rather than absolute absence of energy.

This distinction also removes some of the moral distortion commonly attached to exhaustion. A fatigued person may not lack effort, discipline, desire, or intention. The body may simply be operating under conditions where producing ordinary function has become metabolically expensive.

Tasks feel heavier because they are more expensive relative to current support conditions.

This does not mean the body is permanently damaged whenever fatigue appears. Human physiology is adaptive and dynamic. Utilization cost can rise and fall depending on recovery quality, stress exposure, sleep continuity, illness status, environmental conditions, and broader system stability. The important point is interpretive. Fatigue may represent rising operational expense underneath ordinary function rather than personal inadequacy.

This framework also explains why "trying harder" often fails to fully resolve deep exhaustion. Increased effort may temporarily increase output, but it may simultaneously increase regulatory expense further if underlying strain remains unresolved. The system then spends even more resources preserving continuity while generating less net usable function overall.

Eventually the body responds by narrowing access to output more aggressively because maintaining prior levels has become too costly relative to recoverable capacity.

The body therefore regulates not only fuel availability, but also how expensive it is to transform available fuel into stable output across time.

Understanding fatigue through this lens changes how heaviness, inefficiency, and disproportionate effort are interpreted. The experience is no longer reduced simplistically to motivation, weakness, or lack of desire. Fatigue becomes understandable partly as rising utilization cost under accumulated strain.

The body may still possess fuel. It may still generate energy. But increasing portions of that energy are being redirected toward regulation, repair, adaptation, signaling coordination, stress management, and baseline stability maintenance rather than toward freely accessible output.

Fatigue therefore may emerge not only because fuel access becomes constrained, but because stable function itself becomes increasingly expensive to produce under strain.

And once the cost of producing function is understood, another layer of fatigue becomes easier to recognize. The body must also transition continuously between different fuel states, activity states, and recovery states. Fatigue often becomes especially visible during these transitions when switching between glucose use, fat use, feeding, fasting, rest, and activity demand becomes poorly coordinated.

## Transition Failure Mechanism

Human physiology is not static. The body does not remain in a single fuel state, recovery state, or demand condition continuously across the day. Instead, it moves constantly between changing energetic environments. Feeding transitions into fasting. Rest transitions into activity. Stress activation transitions into recovery. Glucose availability rises and falls. Fuel demands shift according to movement, concentration, emotional load, sleep state, and environmental conditions. Stability therefore depends not only on fuel quantity or total capacity, but also on the ability to transition between states without excessive disruption.

Fatigue often becomes especially visible during these transitions.

The body may appear relatively functional while conditions remain predictable and continuous, yet struggle when rapid adjustment becomes necessary. A person may feel stable immediately after eating but experience heaviness several hours later. Physical activity may begin with unusual sluggishness before function improves. Cognitive performance may deteriorate sharply during periods between meals, after stress exposure, or during abrupt shifts between exertion and recovery. Emotional tolerance may collapse after prolonged activation even when the visible workload itself appears modest.

These experiences frequently reflect transition friction inside the system rather than absolute absence of fuel or total inability to function.

The Transition Failure Mechanism describes this process directly: fatigue can appear when switching between fuel states, activity states, and recovery states becomes delayed, costly, or poorly coordinated.

This mechanism is closely connected to metabolic flexibility, though the focus here is not metabolic flexibility as a standalone concept. The focus is fatigue itself. The body's ability to move between energetic conditions influences whether usable function remains smooth and continuous or becomes unstable and effortful during changing demands.

Transitions themselves carry costs. The body must continually adjust fuel allocation, hormonal signaling, nervous system activity, circulation, glucose availability, tissue uptake, and recovery coordination while demand conditions change. Under stable conditions, these transitions occur with enough efficiency that they remain relatively unnoticed. Under strain, the transitions themselves begin generating fatigue.

This distinction matters because many people interpret fatigue only through stable-state thinking. Energy is imagined as something that either exists or does not exist. In reality, fatigue frequently appears in the space between states rather than entirely inside one state alone.

A person may feel relatively stable during feeding yet fatigued during the transition toward fasting. Another may feel acceptable at rest but unusually heavy during the shift into physical activity. Another may tolerate short-term stress but experience pronounced crashes during attempted recovery afterward. The instability often emerges not because one state is inherently wrong, but because the transition between states becomes poorly coordinated.

Fuel switching is one of the clearest examples. Human physiology continuously alternates between varying degrees of glucose use and fat use depending on timing, activity demand, feeding state, fasting duration, stress conditions, and broader regulatory context. Under flexible conditions, these shifts occur smoothly enough that usable function remains relatively continuous across changing circumstances.

When switching becomes slow, unstable, or inefficient, fatigue often appears during the transition itself.

The body may still contain stored fuel while struggling to access it quickly enough to support current demand. Glucose availability may decline before alternative fuel access becomes sufficiently established. Nervous system stress signaling may rise in response to perceived instability. Concentration may weaken. Irritability increases. Physical heaviness develops. Output becomes inconsistent.

The resulting fatigue frequently feels disproportionate because the body technically still possesses energy reserves. The issue is not total absence. The issue is transition coordination.

This is particularly visible during periods between feeding and fasting states. After eating, incoming fuel and insulin signaling increase nutrient availability and storage coordination. As time passes, the body gradually transitions toward maintaining continuity through stored fuel access, liver glucose release, and broader metabolic adjustment.

When this transition remains smooth, energy continuity is often preserved reasonably well. When the transition becomes strained, the body may temporarily struggle to maintain stable usable fuel access relative to current demand. Fatigue then emerges during the transition zone itself.

The experience may appear as shakiness, heaviness, fog, irritability, unstable concentration, reduced tolerance, or abrupt energy decline. These symptoms often reflect difficulty coordinating fuel accessibility cleanly during changing energetic conditions.

Importantly, this does not mean feeding states are inherently stable or fasting states inherently unstable. Either state can function relatively smoothly or poorly depending on the condition of the system carrying it. The critical variable is coordination.

A stable system transitions without excessive disruption. A strained system experiences friction during change.

Activity demand creates similar transition pressures. The body must rapidly redistribute resources when moving from rest into exertion. Circulation changes. Fuel demand rises. Oxygen delivery increases. Nervous system activation shifts. Muscular coordination intensifies. Hormonal signaling adjusts. Under stable conditions, this transition remains relatively efficient. Under constrained conditions, the transition itself may feel disproportionately exhausting.

A person may therefore experience unusual heaviness at the beginning of activity even when the activity itself is not objectively extreme. The body struggles to shift smoothly into the energetic and regulatory state required to support movement. Output becomes delayed, effortful, or unstable during the transition.

Recovery transitions can become equally difficult. Human physiology is designed not only to activate under stress, but also to downshift afterward. The body must transition from vigilance toward restoration. Heart rate slows. Muscular tension decreases. Stress signaling reduces. Recovery processes intensify. Nervous system activation quiets sufficiently for restorative function to occur effectively.

Under persistent strain, this downshift often becomes impaired.

The body remains partially activated even when external demands decrease. Recovery becomes incomplete because the system cannot fully transition into restorative conditions efficiently. Fatigue then accumulates not only from stress exposure itself, but from difficulty exiting stress states cleanly afterward.

This creates one of the most common patterns in modern fatigue. A person may continue functioning through prolonged activation relatively well while simultaneously becoming increasingly unable to recover effectively afterward. The problem is not merely activation. It is impaired transition out of activation.

The resulting instability frequently appears as restless exhaustion. The person feels tired but unable to fully settle. Sleep becomes shallow or fragmented. Concentration remains strained. Emotional regulation narrows. Recovery periods fail to restore capacity proportionately. The system becomes trapped between activation and restoration without moving smoothly into either state completely.

Poor sleep intensifies transition failure because sleep itself is a major physiological transition. The body must move from wakefulness into restorative regulation. Stress activation must decrease sufficiently. Nervous system signaling must stabilize. Fuel handling must shift appropriately. Repair processes must intensify. When this transition becomes fragmented or incomplete, recovery quality deteriorates even if time in bed remains substantial.

The following day then begins with unresolved strain already present. Subsequent transitions become more expensive because the system is attempting to shift states while carrying accumulated instability from prior cycles.

Recovery debt compounds this process further. The body becomes progressively less adaptable when restoration repeatedly fails to match ongoing demand. Transition flexibility narrows. Small changes in activity, feeding timing, stress load, or sleep continuity begin producing exaggerated fatigue responses because the system possesses less reserve available for adaptation.

Transitions that once felt ordinary now consume disproportionate capacity.

Glucose instability can further increase transition friction because unstable fuel continuity creates abrupt energetic shifts rather than smooth adjustments. Rapid glucose rises followed by steep declines may produce periods where available energy changes faster than the system can comfortably compensate. Stress signaling increases. Irritability rises. Concentration destabilizes. The body experiences the transition itself as strain.

Insulin signaling also influences these transitions because insulin helps coordinate the movement between storage and availability states. Under certain strained conditions, insulin carryover and delayed switching may contribute to periods where glucose accessibility declines before alternative fuel access becomes sufficiently available. The result is not merely low energy, but unstable continuity between energetic states.

Stress load amplifies all of these processes because persistent activation interferes with flexible regulation. The body becomes more rigid under chronic strain. Nervous system signaling remains elevated. Sleep quality deteriorates. Glucose variability increases. Recovery efficiency declines. The system becomes less able to move smoothly between energetic and restorative conditions.

Fatigue then emerges partly because every transition begins carrying higher regulatory expense.

Electrolyte and fluid instability can worsen this friction further because signaling coordination depends on stable gradients and communication efficiency. Muscle contraction, circulatory adjustment, and broader nervous system regulation all rely on these relationships functioning reliably during changing demands. When signaling quality deteriorates, transitions become more effortful and less smooth.

The body therefore experiences change itself as increasingly metabolically expensive.

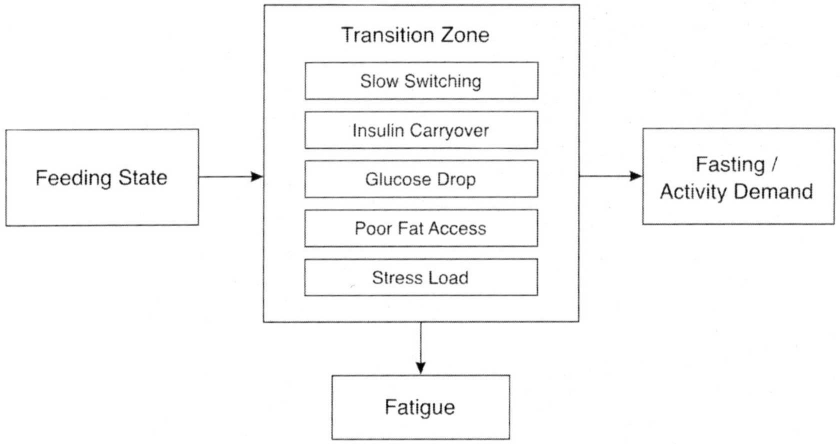


**[Figure 7: Fuel Transition Failure]**

The sequence represented here highlights why fatigue frequently appears in the transition zone itself. Feeding states transition toward fasting and activity demands continuously across ordinary life. Under stable conditions, fuel continuity remains coordinated enough that output stays relatively smooth. Under strained conditions, the transition zone becomes crowded with friction. Slow switching, lingering insulin signaling, glucose instability, poor fat access, and elevated stress load all interfere with clean adaptation. Fatigue then appears not necessarily because fuel disappeared entirely, but because the system struggled to coordinate the shift between states effectively.

This distinction helps explain why some fatigue feels abrupt, unstable, or situational rather than continuously flat. The individual may feel functional in one state and disproportionately fatigued during movement into another. A meal temporarily improves stability before another crash emerges later. Activity feels impossible initially before becoming manageable after adaptation occurs. Stress temporarily increases energy before severe exhaustion appears afterward.

The instability often reflects transition coordination problems rather than singular energy absence.

Importantly, the solution is not perpetual avoidance of transitions. Human physiology depends on flexibility precisely because life continuously changes states. The body must move between feeding and fasting, exertion and recovery, activation and rest. Stability does not mean remaining permanently stimulated, permanently fed, permanently fasted, or permanently inactive.

Stable systems are systems capable of moving between states without excessive disruption.

This distinction matters because fatigue is often interpreted through extremes. Some frameworks attempt to eliminate fatigue through constant stimulation and continuous fuel input. Others attempt to eliminate instability through rigid control of feeding, activity, or recovery conditions. Human physiology is more dynamic than either model allows.

The issue is not that transitions exist. The issue is whether the system can coordinate them efficiently.

Transition failure is therefore one layer within a larger fatigue system rather than a universal explanation for all exhaustion. Sleep quality, stress load, recovery debt, immune strain, fuel availability, utilization cost, and broader load-capacity mismatch all remain deeply relevant. Transition friction simply explains why fatigue often becomes visible during moments of change rather than during stable conditions alone.

This framework also clarifies why fatigue can feel inconsistent. The person is not necessarily imagining variability. Different transitions carry different regulatory demands depending on current system state. A relatively recovered system may transition smoothly through ordinary feeding gaps, activity demands, and recovery periods. A strained system may experience the same transitions as disproportionately destabilizing.

The body therefore reveals instability most clearly during adaptation itself.

This interpretation removes some of the moral confusion surrounding fluctuating fatigue. A person who struggles during transitions is not necessarily weak, lazy, undisciplined, or lacking effort. The system may simply be carrying insufficient flexibility and reserve to coordinate changing demands smoothly under current conditions.

The resulting fatigue often feels uniquely frustrating because function appears unpredictable. Output fluctuates. Energy continuity disappears. Tolerance narrows abruptly. Mental clarity comes and goes. Activity feels accessible temporarily before collapsing unexpectedly afterward.

These patterns frequently reflect instability in coordination rather than absence of desire.

Understanding fatigue through the Transition Failure Mechanism changes the interpretive focus. The body is not simply producing or withholding energy randomly. It is attempting continuously to coordinate fuel states, demand states, and recovery states across changing conditions. When those transitions become delayed, costly, or poorly synchronized, fatigue becomes visible.

The signal therefore deserves contextual interpretation rather than blame. Fatigue often appears during moments when the system cannot move smoothly enough between available fuel, current demand, and restorative conditions to preserve stable usable function across time.

And when transitions repeatedly become more expensive than restoration can offset, another pattern gradually begins emerging underneath the instability itself. Recovery debt accumulates across time as unresolved strain continues carrying forward from one cycle into the next.

# Recovery Debt Mechanism

Fatigue rarely appears only from isolated moments of demand. Human physiology is built to tolerate fluctuation. A poor night of sleep, a difficult week, an intense emotional event, concentrated physical exertion, travel strain, illness recovery, or temporary stress exposure can often be absorbed without producing lasting instability. The body possesses adaptive capacity precisely because life does not unfold under perfectly controlled conditions. Demand rises and falls continuously across ordinary human experience.

The problem emerges when restoration repeatedly fails to fully offset the strain being carried.

Fatigue then begins shifting from an acute response toward an accumulated condition. The body no longer enters each new cycle with restoration substantially complete. Instead, unfinished strain carries forward into the next day, the next week, and eventually the next season of function. Capacity narrows progressively not because one demand was catastrophic, but because restoration repeatedly fell slightly short of what ongoing demand required.

This accumulated shortfall is recovery debt.

The Recovery Debt Mechanism describes this process directly: fatigue can appear when restoration repeatedly falls short of demand, causing unfinished strain to accumulate and reduce available capacity across time.

The important distinction inside this mechanism is that recovery debt is not identical to momentary tiredness. Human beings naturally become tired after exertion, stress, illness, concentration, emotional intensity, or physical work. Acute fatigue is not inherently pathological. In many cases, it reflects normal resource expenditure relative to current demand.

Recovery debt begins when restoration remains incomplete repeatedly enough that unresolved strain becomes cumulative.

This accumulation often develops gradually because small restoration gaps are easy to overlook individually. One shortened night of sleep may feel manageable. One stressful week may seem temporary. One period of increased workload may appear tolerable. One emotionally difficult stretch may feel survivable without obvious collapse.

The body often compensates effectively in the short term. Stress signaling increases alertness. Urgency suppresses awareness of exhaustion. Motivation temporarily preserves output. Additional activation helps maintain visible function despite rising internal cost.

Because compensation remains partially effective, recovery debt frequently develops invisibly at first.

The individual continues functioning outwardly while the system quietly carries increasing amounts of unfinished restoration underneath. Sleep becomes less restorative. Recovery between demands becomes less complete. Emotional resilience narrows. Transition flexibility weakens. Fuel regulation becomes less stable. Stress sensitivity rises. Concentration becomes more effortful. Ordinary tasks consume more of the available stability margin.

The visible workload may remain relatively unchanged while the cost of carrying it rises steadily.

This delayed accumulation is one reason fatigue often feels confusing. People tend to search for immediate causes. Exhaustion appearing today is assumed to originate from today's demands. Physiologically, however, fatigue frequently reflects unresolved strain accumulated across many prior cycles.

The body remembers incomplete restoration.

A useful way to understand recovery debt is through the concept of unfinished restoration. Restoration is not simply inactivity or the absence of work. It is the active rebuilding of support capacity. Nervous system downshifting, tissue repair, hormonal coordination, immune regulation, glucose stabilization, emotional recalibration, fluid balance restoration, and energetic recovery all contribute to rebuilding usable function.

When restoration remains incomplete, the body does not reset fully before new demand arrives.

The next demand is therefore carried by a partially recovered system rather than a fully restored one.

This distinction compounds quickly across time because capacity narrows progressively as unresolved strain accumulates. Early in the process, the reduction may be subtle. Concentration becomes slightly shorter. Patience decreases somewhat. Physical effort feels mildly heavier. Motivation fluctuates more unpredictably. Recovery from exertion becomes slower.

As the debt grows, ordinary demands begin consuming disproportionate capacity.

This is one of the defining experiences of recovery debt. Activities that once felt neutral begin feeling metabolically expensive. Simple responsibilities produce outsized fatigue. Emotional tolerance collapses more rapidly. Cognitive endurance shortens dramatically. Small stressors create exaggerated responses. Recovery from ordinary days begins requiring extraordinary effort.

The visible demand itself often appears insufficient to explain the exhaustion.

This discrepancy leads many people to misinterpret themselves psychologically. They assume reduced function reflects declining motivation, worsening discipline, emotional weakness, aging alone, or insufficient effort. In reality, the system may simply be carrying unresolved restoration deficits accumulated across repeated cycles of under-recovery.

Fatigue then becomes less about today's effort and more about yesterday's unfinished restoration still remaining active inside today's capacity.

The compounding nature of recovery debt is especially important because accumulation is rarely linear. Small restoration gaps do not merely add together mechanically. They often interact with one another. Poor sleep increases stress sensitivity. Elevated stress impairs recovery quality. Recovery impairment destabilizes fuel regulation. Fuel instability increases nervous system strain. Nervous system activation interferes with restorative downshifting. Reduced restoration increases utilization cost further.

The system gradually becomes more expensive to operate while simultaneously possessing less reserve available to absorb new demand.

This interaction helps explain why fatigue often accelerates after long periods of seemingly manageable strain. Compensation masks instability temporarily, but compensation itself consumes resources. Eventually the body can no longer preserve visible function cleanly. Ordinary demands then begin triggering disproportionate exhaustion because the accumulated recovery debt has narrowed the stability margin too far.

Importantly, recovery debt does not always announce itself immediately after the demand that produced it. Fatigue is often delayed. A person may function relatively well during a stressful period, major project, travel sequence, caregiving demand, illness response, or emotionally intense season while simultaneously accumulating unresolved strain underneath.

The exhaustion sometimes appears afterward rather than during the event itself.

This delayed fatigue confuses interpretation because people expect strain and exhaustion to occur simultaneously. Physiologically, however, activation can temporarily suppress awareness of depletion. Stress hormones increase vigilance and short-term output. Urgency focuses attention externally. Social or professional pressure sustains performance temporarily.

When the activating conditions finally decrease, the accumulated restoration deficit becomes more visible. The body no longer needs to suppress fatigue signals to preserve immediate function. The unresolved debt then surfaces more clearly.

This is why people often "crash" after prolonged periods of sustained demand rather than during them.

The crash is rarely random. It reflects accumulated unfinished restoration becoming impossible to continue masking effectively.

Recovery debt also explains why some fatigue feels heavy rather than unstable. Earlier mechanisms involved fuel accessibility, transition friction, or rising utilization cost. Recovery debt adds another layer: accumulated reduction in baseline capacity itself. The body is no longer operating from full reserve. Every activity begins closer to the system's remaining limit.

The resulting fatigue often feels dense, persistent, and disproportionate to visible effort because the system is carrying unresolved strain continuously in the background.

Stress load interacts with this process constantly. Persistent stress activation interferes with complete restoration because the body struggles to fully downshift into recovery states while vigilance remains elevated. Nervous system signaling stays partially activated. Sleep becomes lighter or more fragmented. Emotional processing remains incomplete. Muscular tension persists. Recovery efficiency declines.

The body then accumulates restoration gaps even if outward activity levels appear moderate.

Poor sleep amplifies this accumulation further because sleep quality influences nearly every restorative process involved in rebuilding capacity. Sleep disruption does not merely create temporary tiredness. Repeated sleep disruption increases regulation cost, destabilizes fuel continuity, impairs emotional tolerance, raises stress sensitivity, weakens transition flexibility, and narrows the stability margin available for future demand.

The resulting fatigue therefore reflects accumulation rather than isolated depletion.

Fuel availability interacts with recovery debt as well. A strained system often handles energetic transitions less efficiently. Glucose stability may worsen. Stress signaling may rise more easily during fuel gaps. Metabolic flexibility may narrow. Energy continuity becomes harder to maintain because the body is attempting to regulate fuel while already carrying unresolved restoration deficits.

Utilization cost rises simultaneously. More energy is spent maintaining baseline stability and compensation, leaving less net usable function available for discretionary output.

The body therefore enters a progressively more constrained state where restoration becomes harder precisely because strain has already accumulated.

This compounding process explains why recovery debt frequently remains hidden while visible functioning continues outwardly. Many people assume that preserved performance proves adequate recovery. Physiology does not necessarily work that way. Human beings can continue producing output for long periods through compensation while accumulating significant unresolved strain underneath.

The eventual fatigue then appears disproportionate because the visible workload alone seems too small to explain the collapse.

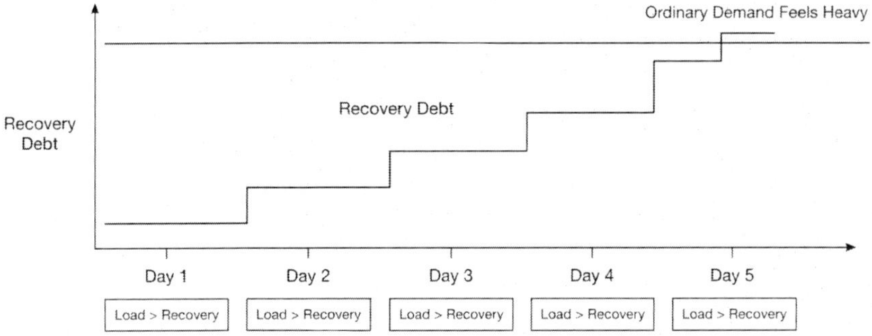


**[Figure 8: Recovery Debt Accumulation]**

The pattern represented here clarifies why fatigue often emerges gradually rather than suddenly. Small restoration gaps repeat across multiple cycles. Load continues exceeding recovery by seemingly manageable amounts. The debt line rises incrementally at first, often unnoticed because compensation preserves function. Eventually the accumulated debt crosses a threshold where ordinary demands begin feeling unusually heavy. The fatigue signal then becomes more visible not because the person suddenly weakened, but because unfinished restoration has progressively narrowed available capacity across time.

This accumulated narrowing affects nearly every aspect of function. Concentration becomes less stable because cognitive effort consumes more of the reduced reserve. Physical exertion feels heavier because recovery capacity remains incomplete. Emotional tolerance narrows because stress buffering requires resources the system no longer possesses comfortably. Motivation fluctuates because initiation itself becomes metabolically expensive under constrained conditions. Fuel regulation destabilizes because energetic coordination is occurring within an already strained environment.

Even ordinary transitions become more difficult because flexibility depends partly on reserve capacity.

Recovery debt therefore influences the entire system rather than one isolated symptom.

Importantly, this mechanism should not become a universal explanation for all fatigue. Human exhaustion remains multi-layered. Illness, acute stress, immune strain, fuel instability, transition friction, utilization cost, and broader load-capacity mismatch all contribute meaningfully to different fatigue experiences. Recovery debt is central because accumulation shapes long-term stability profoundly, but it does not erase the importance of other mechanisms.

The important shift is interpretive. Fatigue often reflects unfinished restoration carried forward across time rather than sudden weakness or insufficient effort.

This interpretation removes some of the moral distortion attached to exhaustion. A person carrying substantial recovery debt may appear functional externally while internally operating with dramatically narrowed reserve. The body is not necessarily refusing effort irrationally. It is attempting to preserve continuity under accumulated unresolved strain.

The resulting fatigue is therefore not merely laziness, fragility, or lack of motivation. It is often the experiential cost of carrying unfinished restoration across too many repeated cycles without adequate rebuilding of support capacity.

This also explains why recovery sometimes feels slower than expected once exhaustion becomes severe. The body is not merely restoring today's strain. It may be attempting to repay accumulated restoration deficits built across weeks, months, or longer periods of under-recovery. Capacity rebuilding takes time because the debt itself accumulated gradually.

The goal is therefore not eliminating all demand from human life. Demand is normal. Challenge, exertion, emotional intensity, cognitive effort, and adaptation are all part of healthy human function. Stability does not require perfect comfort or perpetual rest.

Stable systems are systems where restoration and demand remain sufficiently aligned across time that unfinished strain does not accumulate faster than recovery can resolve it.

When that alignment deteriorates repeatedly, recovery debt rises quietly underneath visible life. Ordinary tasks become heavier. Stress responses intensify. Output narrows. Fatigue becomes more persistent because the system is no longer functioning from restored capacity.

The fatigue signal then reflects accumulation rather than isolated depletion.

And once recovery debt is understood as unfinished restoration carried across repeated cycles, another important distinction begins emerging underneath the idea of recovery itself. Time spent asleep is not automatically identical to restoration. Sleep duration alone does not guarantee that the processes required to rebuild capacity are occurring effectively enough to fully restore the system.

# Sleep-Recovery Translation Mechanism

Sleep is often treated as the body's universal reset mechanism, but fatigue frequently reveals a more complicated reality. A person may spend substantial time asleep and still wake feeling heavy, foggy, strained, unrestored, or disproportionately fatigued relative to the apparent amount of rest obtained. This experience creates confusion because sleep duration is commonly interpreted as interchangeable with recovery itself. Physiologically, however, time spent asleep and restoration achieved during sleep are related but distinct conditions.

Sleep is a major recovery input. It is not an automatic guarantee of complete restoration.

The body does not rebuild capacity merely because unconsciousness occurred for a certain number of hours. Recovery depends on whether sleep successfully translates into nervous system downshifting, hormonal coordination, tissue restoration, metabolic recalibration, immune regulation, emotional processing, and broader rebuilding of usable function across systems.

The Sleep-Recovery Translation Mechanism describes this directly: fatigue can persist when time spent asleep does not translate fully into restoration, capacity rebuilding, and nervous system downshifting.

This distinction matters because many experiences of fatigue involve incomplete recovery translation rather than simple absence of sleep opportunity. A person may technically sleep long enough while still failing to obtain the depth, continuity, regulation quality, or restorative coordination necessary to meaningfully rebuild capacity.

The resulting fatigue often feels especially frustrating because the visible recovery behavior appears correct. Time was spent in bed. Sleep occurred. Yet usable function remains constrained.

This mismatch between sleep quantity and recovery effect leads many people to interpret themselves negatively. Persistent fatigue after sleep is often framed as laziness, lack of discipline, low motivation, aging alone, or personal weakness because sleep duration is assumed to guarantee restoration automatically.

Human physiology operates more dynamically than that.

Recovery is not merely passive unconsciousness. It is an active regulatory process. Nervous system signaling must shift away from sustained activation. Hormonal rhythms must coordinate appropriately. Tissue repair processes intensify. Energy restoration occurs. Immune activity recalibrates. Stress signaling decreases sufficiently for restorative function to become dominant rather than defensive.

Sleep provides the opportunity for these processes. Whether the opportunity translates successfully into recovery depends on the condition of the system entering sleep and the quality of the restorative state achieved during it.

This distinction becomes especially visible under prolonged stress. A person may sleep for substantial periods while remaining physiologically activated underneath. Nervous system strain persists. Muscular tension remains elevated. Stress signaling continues. Emotional vigilance remains partially active. Sleep occurs, but full downshifting does not.

The body therefore spends much of the sleep period maintaining activation rather than fully transitioning into restoration.

The resulting fatigue often feels paradoxical because the individual technically slept. Yet the system never fully entered deep restorative coordination consistently enough to rebuild capacity proportionately.

This is one reason sleep quality matters independently from sleep duration. Fragmented sleep, unstable sleep architecture, repeated awakenings, shallow recovery depth, disrupted timing, inconsistent circadian alignment, or prolonged stress activation can all interfere with the translation from sleep time into actual restoration.

The body may therefore spend many hours asleep while rebuilding far less usable function than expected.

A useful distinction exists between sleep exposure and recovery effect. Sleep exposure refers to time spent asleep or attempting sleep. Recovery effect refers to the actual rebuilding of capacity achieved through that sleep. The two frequently overlap, but they are not identical.

Under stable conditions, sleep exposure often produces substantial recovery effect. Under strained conditions, the translation becomes less efficient.

This inefficiency helps explain why recovery debt can continue accumulating even when sleep duration appears outwardly reasonable. The body may receive sleep opportunity repeatedly while still failing to fully restore nervous system balance, emotional resilience, metabolic stability, immune recovery, and energetic continuity.

The restoration gap remains active underneath the counted hours.

Stress load plays a major role in this process because stress alters the body's ability to fully transition into restorative states. Acute stress can temporarily suppress fatigue awareness by increasing vigilance and activation. Persistent stress exposure often interferes with restorative depth afterward. Sleep becomes lighter, more fragmented, or less restorative even when duration remains relatively intact.

The body struggles to fully release activation because the system continues prioritizing vigilance.

This persistent activation changes how sleep feels subjectively and how restoration unfolds physiologically. A person may wake feeling unrefreshed not because sleep never occurred, but because the body remained partially engaged in stress regulation throughout the night rather than fully reallocating resources toward recovery.

Emotional load contributes similarly. Human physiology does not separate emotional strain cleanly from recovery quality. Ongoing uncertainty, unresolved tension, grief, anticipation, vigilance, conflict, and emotional processing all influence nervous system state entering sleep. The body carries these regulatory demands into the restorative period itself.

Sleep then becomes less efficient at rebuilding capacity because portions of the system remain occupied with ongoing regulation and adaptation.

Glucose instability can interfere with recovery translation through different pathways. Stable restorative function depends partly on stable overnight fuel coordination. Large fluctuations in glucose availability, stress-related hormonal shifts, or unstable metabolic regulation may increase nighttime activation, reduce continuity of restorative depth, or disrupt the body's ability to remain physiologically stable throughout sleep.

The resulting fatigue often feels disproportionate because the issue is not only reduced sleep quantity. It is unstable restoration quality underneath the duration.

Immune strain also alters sleep-recovery translation substantially. During illness recovery or periods of elevated immune activity, the body reallocates resources toward repair, defense, and restoration. Sleep demand may increase while subjective restoration remains incomplete because the system is carrying substantial internal regulatory burden continuously.

A person may therefore sleep longer than usual while still feeling fatigued because the body is directing large portions of available recovery toward internal maintenance rather than toward rebuilding discretionary capacity fully.

This distinction matters because fatigue after sleep does not automatically indicate failure, weakness, or insufficient effort. The body may simply be operating under conditions where restoration efficiency has become impaired relative to current demand.

Poor sleep translation also explains why some forms of fatigue feel qualitatively different from simple sleepiness. Sleepiness reflects immediate drive toward sleep. Under-recovery often feels broader. Concentration weakens. Emotional tolerance narrows. Physical heaviness persists. Motivation fluctuates. Cognitive continuity deteriorates. Recovery from ordinary activity slows.

The person may not merely want more sleep. The system may require more complete restoration than current sleep conditions are providing.

Circadian alignment influences this process because restorative function unfolds within broader biological timing patterns. Hormonal rhythms, temperature regulation, nervous system cycling, metabolic coordination, and sleep depth all interact with timing consistency across repeated cycles. When timing becomes highly disrupted or physiologically misaligned, sleep may occur without translating fully into stable recovery.

This does not mean human physiology requires perfection. The body is adaptive and capable of tolerating variability. Problems emerge primarily when disruption becomes prolonged enough that restoration repeatedly fails to rebuild capacity proportionately across time.

The resulting fatigue often appears gradual because incomplete restoration accumulates quietly before becoming obvious.

This accumulation closely connects to recovery debt. Recovery debt is not merely caused by sleeping less. It can also develop when sleep repeatedly fails to produce sufficient recovery effect relative to current load. A person may therefore carry substantial under-recovery despite spending significant time asleep because the translation from sleep into restoration remains incomplete.

The body remembers ineffective restoration just as it remembers insufficient restoration.

This is one reason fatigue often persists after apparently "catching up" on sleep. Time asleep may increase temporarily while deeper recovery processes remain slower to rebuild. Nervous system activation may still remain elevated. Emotional strain may still remain unresolved. Metabolic regulation may still remain unstable. Immune recovery may still remain incomplete.

The visible sleep behavior changes faster than the underlying restoration state.

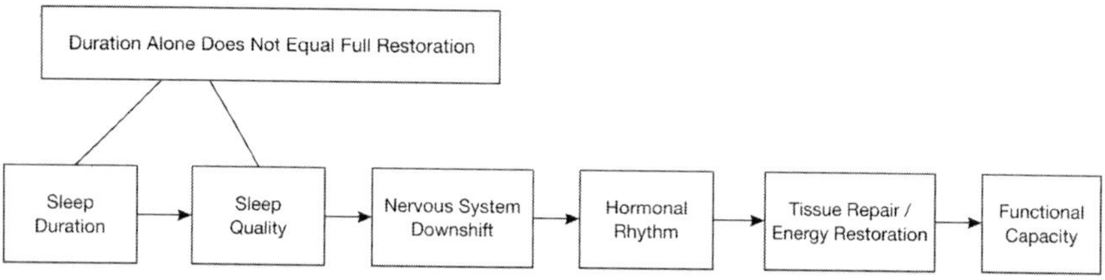


**[Figure 9: Sleep-to-Recovery Translation]**

The pathway represented here clarifies why sleep duration alone cannot fully explain recovery quality. Sleep time provides the starting condition, but restoration depends on what happens physiologically during that period. Sleep quality, nervous system downshifting, hormonal rhythm coordination, tissue repair, and energy restoration all influence whether usable functional capacity is actually rebuilt. The side note matters because it separates counted hours from restorative effect. Duration alone does not guarantee full recovery translation.

This distinction also explains why sleep can restore certain systems while leaving others relatively strained. Physical heaviness may improve while emotional tolerance remains narrow. Cognitive sharpness may partially recover while stress sensitivity remains elevated. Sleep is not a single on-off process affecting every domain equally. Restoration unfolds across interacting systems with different demands and different recovery timelines.

The body therefore may feel partially restored and partially depleted simultaneously.

This layered recovery pattern often confuses people because fatigue is expected to disappear cleanly once enough sleep occurs. Human restoration is more distributed than that. Different systems recover at different speeds depending on prior strain, current load, immune activity, emotional burden, stress state, fuel regulation, and nervous system conditions entering sleep itself.

The resulting fatigue may therefore linger even after sleep duration improves because the deeper restoration processes remain incomplete.

Importantly, this chapter should not be interpreted as minimizing the importance of sleep duration. Severe or chronic sleep restriction profoundly affects fatigue stability. Time asleep matters enormously because restoration requires opportunity. The distinction is simply that opportunity and outcome are not always interchangeable.

The body requires sleep exposure in order to rebuild capacity, but sleep exposure alone does not guarantee the rebuilding occurred fully.

This framework also avoids reducing sleep to optimization culture. Human beings are not machines requiring perfect nightly metrics in order to function acceptably. The body is adaptive. Variability exists naturally across ordinary life. One poor night of sleep, one disrupted schedule, one stressful period, or one fragmented cycle does not automatically produce collapse.

The concern emerges when incomplete restoration becomes repeated and cumulative across time.

Persistent or severe unrefreshing sleep also deserves careful attention rather than dismissal. Fatigue that remains profound despite adequate sleep opportunity should not automatically be minimized as laziness or lack of effort. Many factors can interfere with restorative translation, and persistent disruption may warrant appropriate evaluation. The important distinction here is interpretive rather than diagnostic. The presence of fatigue after sleep does not inherently reveal moral failure or personal inadequacy.

It may instead reflect incomplete recovery translation underneath the sleep itself.

This understanding changes how fatigue after sleep is interpreted psychologically. The individual is not necessarily unwilling, weak, or undisciplined simply because rest failed to restore function proportionately. The body may be struggling to convert sleep exposure into meaningful capacity rebuilding under current conditions.

That struggle often reflects interaction among stress load, emotional strain, nervous system activation, metabolic instability, immune burden, recovery debt, and broader system regulation.

The resulting fatigue is therefore not merely about sleep quantity. It is about restoration quality and recovery translation.

This distinction also explains why stimulation frequently fails to resolve deep exhaustion cleanly after poor recovery translation. Increased activation can temporarily increase alertness while leaving the underlying restoration deficit unchanged. The person may feel briefly more awake while remaining fundamentally under-recovered underneath.

The system still lacks rebuilt reserve.

Sleep therefore matters not simply because unconscious time occurred, but because the body must successfully transition that time into restoration, nervous system downshifting, tissue rebuilding, metabolic recalibration, and recovered usable function.

When this translation becomes impaired, fatigue persists despite apparent rest because restoration remains incomplete beneath the duration itself.

And once sleep is understood as a recovery input rather than an automatic recovery outcome, another pattern becomes easier to recognize. Even after the obvious stressor ends or sleep finally occurs, restoration itself may lag behind demand, leaving fatigue present long after the visible cause appears to have passed.

# Restoration Lag Mechanism

Fatigue is often expected to disappear once the obvious demand ends. A stressful project concludes. Travel stops. Illness resolves. Workload decreases. Sleep improves for several nights. Emotional conflict settles. Training intensity falls. The visible stressor recedes, yet fatigue frequently remains present long afterward. This persistence creates confusion because recovery is commonly imagined as immediate. Once demand decreases, restored capacity is expected to return automatically and proportionately.

Human physiology rarely operates that quickly.

The body does not reset instantly when stress ends. Reduced load and restored capacity are not the same event. External conditions can improve rapidly while internal restoration continues unfolding much more slowly underneath. Fatigue may therefore persist not because the body failed irrationally, but because recovery itself requires time, coordination, and ongoing rebuilding after the visible demand has already passed.

This delay is restoration lag.

The Restoration Lag Mechanism describes this directly: fatigue can persist when external demand decreases faster than internal capacity is restored.

This distinction matters because many forms of lingering fatigue are interpreted psychologically rather than physiologically. A person expects relief after the stressor disappears. When exhaustion remains, the experience is often interpreted as weakness, laziness, low resilience, poor motivation, or inability to "move on." In reality, the system may still be carrying unresolved restoration processes long after the visible trigger has ended.

The body remembers strain beyond the moment of exposure itself.

A useful way to understand restoration lag is through the difference between stopping damage and rebuilding capacity. Removing or reducing a demand changes the environment surrounding the system. Restoration requires the system itself to recover afterward. Those processes overlap, but they are not identical.

A stressful month ending does not instantly normalize nervous system regulation. Several nights of improved sleep do not automatically erase accumulated recovery debt. Illness resolution does not mean tissue repair and immune recalibration finished simultaneously with symptom reduction. Reduced workload does not immediately restore emotional resilience, fuel stability, concentration, and physical endurance.

The visible demand often disappears before the underlying restoration process completes.

This lag is especially apparent after prolonged activation. Human physiology can sustain heightened alertness, stress adaptation, concentrated output, emotional vigilance, and temporary compensation for surprisingly long periods. During those periods, fatigue signals are often partially suppressed because maintaining function remains necessary. Stress signaling helps preserve output. Urgency increases focus temporarily. Adrenal activation narrows attention toward immediate demands.

Once the stressor ends, however, the body no longer needs to maintain the same level of activation. The accumulated strain then becomes more visible because suppression decreases.

This is one reason people frequently feel more exhausted after the demanding period ends rather than during it.

The fatigue is not newly created after the stressor. It was already accumulating underneath the activation state. The end of the stressor simply allowed the body to stop prioritizing immediate performance over awareness of strain.

This delayed fatigue confuses interpretation because people expect relief to feel immediate. Instead, the nervous system often remains partially activated long after the visible demand decreases. Stress signaling does not disappear instantly. Sleep quality may remain unstable. Emotional vigilance may persist. Recovery depth may remain incomplete. Fuel regulation may still carry instability produced during the earlier strain period.

The body therefore continues operating under elevated regulation cost even though the original stressor has technically ended.

Recovery debt amplifies this lag significantly. Accumulated under-recovery narrows available capacity progressively across time. When the demand period finally decreases, the body still carries unresolved restoration deficits built during the earlier strain. Capacity rebuilding unfolds gradually because restoration itself requires resources, coordination, and time.

The resulting fatigue often feels disproportionate because current visible demands appear relatively modest compared to the exhaustion being experienced. The person may wonder why ordinary activities still feel heavy after the difficult period supposedly ended.

Physiologically, the answer is often that capacity has not yet fully rebuilt.

The body may still be recalibrating sleep architecture, restoring emotional tolerance, stabilizing fuel continuity, reducing stress signaling, repairing tissue strain, resolving immune activation, and rebuilding broader support capacity underneath visible daily life.

This process frequently unfolds more slowly than people expect because restoration is not a switch. It is a layered progression.

Some systems recover faster than others. Acute stress activation may decrease relatively quickly while emotional resilience remains narrow. Sleep duration may improve before sleep-recovery translation fully stabilizes. Physical energy may partially return while concentration remains fragile. Immune strain may decrease while nervous system activation remains elevated.

The body therefore may feel simultaneously improved and under-recovered at the same time.

This layered recovery pattern explains why temporary relief does not always equal full restoration. A person may experience several better days and assume recovery is complete, only to encounter disproportionate fatigue again under relatively ordinary demand. The system had improved partially but had not yet fully rebuilt reserve capacity.

The stability margin remained narrower than expected.

Travel strain illustrates this process clearly. Long travel periods often disrupt sleep timing, circadian alignment, meal timing, nervous system regulation, hydration continuity, and broader recovery coordination simultaneously. The travel itself eventually ends, but the body may continue carrying disrupted rhythms and elevated regulation cost afterward.

Fatigue then lingers because the internal system has not yet fully reorganized into stable recovery patterns.

Illness recovery behaves similarly. Visible symptoms may improve substantially before restoration fully completes underneath. Immune strain, tissue repair, nervous system recalibration, sleep normalization, and energetic rebuilding often continue after the obvious illness phase appears finished.

The resulting lingering fatigue frequently confuses people because they assume symptom reduction and restored capacity should occur simultaneously.

Human recovery unfolds more gradually than that.

The same pattern appears after prolonged emotional strain. Conflict resolves. A stressful situation stabilizes. Uncertainty decreases. Yet the body may remain fatigued for extended periods afterward because nervous system signaling, sleep disruption, emotional vigilance, and accumulated recovery debt continue operating underneath the apparent resolution.

The body often exits the stressful environment before it exits the physiological stress state fully.

This distinction is important because lingering fatigue is frequently moralized unnecessarily. When exhaustion persists after visible demands decrease, people often assume they are failing to recover correctly. They criticize themselves for remaining tired despite supposedly having less reason to feel that way.

Physiology is not obligated to restore capacity on the same timeline that external conditions improve.

The nervous system requires time to fully downshift after prolonged activation. Sleep quality often normalizes gradually rather than instantly. Fuel stability may remain fragile for a period after major stress exposure. Emotional tolerance rebuilds progressively. Recovery debt repays incrementally. Capacity restoration unfolds through process rather than through immediate reversal.

The body therefore may continue signaling fatigue long after the visible demand itself has disappeared.

This does not mean all lingering fatigue should automatically be normalized or ignored indefinitely. Persistent, severe, worsening, or unexplained fatigue deserves appropriate attention rather than dismissal. The important distinction is interpretive. Fatigue after stress or strain does not automatically imply weakness, laziness, or personal inadequacy simply because the visible stressor ended already.

Restoration may still be underway underneath the current experience.

Sleep-recovery translation strongly influences restoration lag because sleep opportunity alone does not guarantee immediate rebuilding of capacity. A person may begin sleeping longer after a stressful period while still remaining physiologically under-recovered. Nervous system activation may still interfere with deep restoration. Emotional processing may still remain active. Fuel regulation may still require recalibration. Recovery depth may still remain incomplete.

The visible sleep improvement therefore occurs before the deeper recovery effect fully catches up.

Stress load compounds this lag because prolonged activation changes baseline regulation itself. The body adapts to vigilance during high-demand periods. Returning from that activated state often takes time even after external conditions improve. The system must relearn downshifting rather than remaining prepared continuously for further strain.

This recalibration period frequently feels uncomfortable because activation and exhaustion coexist simultaneously. The person feels tired but restless, depleted yet unable to fully settle. Sleep improves somewhat but not completely. Recovery occurs, but more slowly than expected.

The body is transitioning gradually out of prolonged stress adaptation.

Fuel stability also influences restoration lag because prolonged strain often disrupts energetic continuity. Stress signaling alters glucose regulation. Sleep disruption changes appetite and fuel handling. Nervous system activation increases energetic instability. When the stressor ends, these patterns may persist temporarily before broader coordination stabilizes again.

The resulting fatigue reflects ongoing recalibration rather than ongoing visible stress exposure.

Immune strain behaves similarly. The body may continue allocating resources toward repair and restoration after the most visible symptoms have resolved. Fatigue then persists partly because significant internal recovery work is still underway even though the person appears outwardly improved.

The system is rebuilding capacity underneath reduced visible demand.

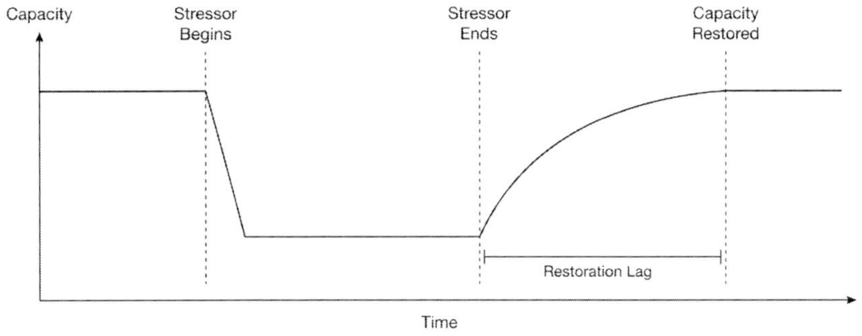


**[Figure 10: Restoration Lag Curve]**

The relationship represented here clarifies why fatigue often lingers after obvious stressors end. Capacity drops during periods of elevated demand, prolonged activation, illness, disrupted sleep, emotional strain, or accumulated recovery debt. When the stressor finally decreases, capacity does not immediately return to baseline. Instead, restoration unfolds gradually across time. The gap between the end of the stressor and the rebuilding of capacity is restoration lag. Fatigue remains present during this gap not because the body failed to recover instantly, but because restoration itself requires ongoing rebuilding after the visible demand has already decreased.

This framework changes how delayed fatigue is interpreted. The person is not necessarily becoming weaker after the difficult period. In many cases, the body is finally allowing accumulated strain to become visible now that immediate performance demands have decreased. The fatigue signal reflects unresolved restoration rather than sudden collapse.

This distinction also explains why some individuals function surprisingly well during intense periods yet deteriorate afterward. Activation temporarily preserved output. Recovery processes were postponed or incomplete. Once the pressure eased, the unresolved strain became harder to continue suppressing.

The exhaustion therefore reflects accumulated restoration cost surfacing after the demand period rather than emotional fragility or lack of discipline.

Importantly, restoration lag is one mechanism inside a larger fatigue system rather than a universal explanation for every exhaustion pattern. Fuel instability, recovery debt, immune strain, sleep disruption, transition friction, rising utilization cost, and broader load-capacity mismatch all remain deeply relevant. Restoration lag simply explains why fatigue often persists after the visible demand appears to have resolved already.

The body rebuilds more slowly than many external demands disappear.

This understanding also restores proportionality to recovery expectations. Human physiology is adaptive but not instantaneous. Capacity rebuilding unfolds across overlapping processes involving nervous system regulation, sleep-recovery translation, energetic stabilization, emotional recalibration, tissue restoration, and broader support recovery. These processes operate across time rather than through immediate reset.

The body therefore deserves interpretation rather than accusation when lingering fatigue remains present after strain.

Fatigue in these situations often reflects the time required for restoration to catch up to the earlier demand that reduced capacity in the first place.

And once restoration lag is understood, another important layer of fatigue becomes more visible underneath ongoing strain itself. Stress load is not merely emotional discomfort or mental pressure. Vigilance, uncertainty, conflict, emotional demand, decision burden, and continuous adaptation all carry substantial regulation cost that consumes usable capacity across time.

# Stress Load Mechanism

Stress is often interpreted as an emotional experience, but fatigue reveals a broader physiological reality. The body does not distinguish sharply between emotional demand, environmental pressure, cognitive burden, uncertainty, vigilance, conflict, adaptation, and physical strain. All of these conditions require allocation. Resources must be redirected. Attention must be maintained. Nervous system signaling must remain coordinated. Sleep quality changes. Fuel regulation shifts. Emotional tolerance narrows. Recovery processes become more difficult to complete fully.

Stress therefore functions not merely as a feeling, but as continuous physiological coordination under perceived demand.

This distinction matters because fatigue associated with stress is frequently misunderstood. People often search for visible exertion to justify exhaustion. If there was no intense physical activity, the fatigue may appear illegitimate or exaggerated. A person may spend much of the day sitting, thinking, worrying, anticipating, caregiving, negotiating conflict, navigating uncertainty, making decisions, suppressing emotional reactions, or remaining continuously vigilant while appearing externally inactive.

Physiologically, the body may still be carrying enormous load.

The Stress Load Mechanism describes this directly: fatigue can emerge when sustained stress, vigilance, uncertainty, emotional demand, and continuous adaptation increase the regulatory cost required to maintain stable function across time.

The important concept inside this mechanism is regulation cost. Human physiology must continuously coordinate internal stability under changing conditions. The nervous system monitors safety, uncertainty, environmental demand, social tension, physical strain, fuel continuity, emotional salience, and anticipated threat continuously. Under stable conditions, much of this coordination remains efficient enough that it stays relatively invisible.

Under sustained stress exposure, the cost of maintaining that coordination rises progressively.

This increased cost explains why stress frequently produces physical fatigue even without substantial visible exertion. The body is not merely "thinking too much." It is reallocating resources toward vigilance, adaptation, prediction, emotional regulation, and continuity maintenance across systems simultaneously.

The experience often feels physical because it is physical.

Muscular tension increases. Sleep becomes lighter or more fragmented. Fuel regulation becomes less stable. Recovery depth decreases. Concentration consumes more effort. Emotional regulation becomes metabolically expensive. Ordinary decisions require disproportionate energy. The body begins operating under sustained activation rather than under efficient restoration.

This activation is not inherently pathological. Stress signaling exists because adaptation is necessary for survival. Cortisol and nervous system activation are not enemies of physiology. They help preserve continuity under immediate demand. Acute stress can increase alertness, sharpen attention, mobilize fuel, and temporarily support performance during periods requiring rapid adaptation.

The body is designed to respond dynamically when circumstances demand increased vigilance or effort.

Problems emerge primarily when activation persists long enough that restoration repeatedly becomes incomplete.

The body then shifts from temporary adaptive mobilization into elevated baseline operating cost.

This shift is gradual enough that many people fail to recognize it while it is occurring. Stress often becomes normalized internally before fatigue becomes unmistakable externally. A person adapts to constant deadlines, uncertainty, emotional suppression, caregiving burden, financial instability, conflict, social tension, cognitive overload, or prolonged anticipation by carrying increasing levels of activation continuously.

The system compensates remarkably well at first. Output remains possible. Responsibilities continue. Concentration appears intact externally. The body preserves continuity through increased regulation effort.

Underneath that preserved function, however, recovery efficiency frequently declines.

Sleep becomes less restorative because nervous system downshifting remains incomplete. Emotional regulation consumes more energy because baseline vigilance remains elevated. Fuel stability becomes more variable because stress signaling continuously alters metabolic coordination. Recovery debt accumulates because restoration repeatedly falls short of the regulation cost required to maintain adaptation.

Fatigue then emerges partly because the body is spending increasing amounts of energy preserving stability itself.

This distinction is essential because stress-related fatigue is often moralized incorrectly. A person carrying significant invisible load may appear physically inactive while internally functioning under extreme regulatory demand. Others may interpret the exhaustion as overreaction because the workload is not visibly physical.

The body responds to total load, not merely visible movement.

Decision burden alone can become metabolically expensive under sustained conditions. Every unresolved choice, conflict, uncertainty, responsibility, interruption, and anticipated outcome requires ongoing regulation. Cognitive load is not weightless. Emotional suppression is not free. Social vigilance consumes resources. Caregiving strain demands continuous attentional allocation even during periods that appear externally quiet.

The nervous system continuously evaluates uncertainty and potential disruption because prediction itself helps preserve stability. Under prolonged uncertainty, the body remains partially activated because resolution never fully arrives. The system continues preparing, monitoring, anticipating, and adapting without fully downshifting into restoration.

Fatigue then accumulates because the body is paying the energetic cost of vigilance continuously.

This helps explain why stress frequently produces heaviness rather than simple emotional discomfort. The body becomes physically burdened because regulation itself consumes resources. Concentration feels dense. Physical movement becomes effortful. Emotional tolerance narrows. Ordinary tasks begin feeling disproportionately expensive. Recovery periods no longer fully restore capacity.

The person may assume they simply lack motivation. Physiologically, the system may be carrying sustained adaptation cost underneath every ordinary action.

A major source of confusion is that acute stress can temporarily preserve output extremely effectively. During periods of immediate demand, the body increases activation in order to maintain function. Attention sharpens. Fuel mobilization increases. Fatigue awareness may decrease temporarily. The person often performs adequately during the stressful event itself.

The exhaustion frequently appears afterward.

This delayed fatigue is not contradictory. The body prioritized immediate adaptation over restoration during the demand period. Once the activating conditions decrease, the accumulated regulation cost becomes harder to suppress. Fatigue surfaces because the system no longer needs to preserve short-term output at the same intensity.

This is why people often experience crashes after prolonged work strain, caregiving periods, emotional conflict, travel, crisis management, or sustained uncertainty. The fatigue was not absent during the stress period. It was partially masked through activation.

The body eventually begins revealing the accumulated cost of maintaining adaptation continuously.

Stress also interacts heavily with fuel regulation. Sustained activation changes how the body mobilizes and distributes energy. Cortisol and broader stress signaling influence glucose availability, insulin coordination, appetite regulation, and fuel continuity across time. Under prolonged stress exposure, energy stability often becomes less predictable.

A person may experience periods of temporary alertness followed by abrupt heaviness, fog, irritability, shakiness, or reduced tolerance. Fuel continuity becomes unstable partly because the body is repeatedly reallocating resources under ongoing perceived demand.

This instability further increases regulation cost because maintaining energetic continuity itself becomes more difficult.

Sleep quality deteriorates simultaneously. Even when sleep duration appears relatively adequate, nervous system activation may prevent full downshifting into deep restorative states. Sleep becomes lighter, more fragmented, or less restorative. The body remains partially prepared for demand even during the recovery period itself.

Recovery debt then accumulates because restoration repeatedly fails to fully offset the cost of ongoing vigilance.

This interaction creates a compounding effect. Stress increases regulation expense. Reduced restoration decreases available capacity. Reduced capacity increases stress sensitivity. Increased sensitivity raises activation further. Fuel instability worsens. Emotional tolerance narrows.

Ordinary demands begin consuming larger percentages of the remaining reserve.

Fatigue then becomes progressively more visible because the body is carrying rising operational cost underneath ordinary life.

Importantly, stress is not limited to dramatic crisis. Many forms of stress are quiet, prolonged, and socially normalized. Persistent uncertainty, emotional suppression, unresolved conflict, anticipatory anxiety, caregiving responsibility, financial instability, constant interruption, social vigilance, environmental overstimulation, and continuous low-level pressure can all produce significant physiological load across time.

The invisibility of these demands often makes the resulting fatigue difficult for people to validate internally. The person may feel exhausted while simultaneously believing they have not "done enough" to justify the exhaustion.

Physiology does not require visible physical collapse in order to accumulate strain.

The body responds to coordination demand itself.

This explains why stress can make ordinary tasks feel metabolically expensive. The task is no longer occurring inside a rested, stable, flexible system. It is occurring inside a system already spending substantial resources maintaining vigilance and adaptation. Every additional action therefore consumes proportionately more of the remaining reserve.

Concentration becomes effortful because attention regulation is already strained. Emotional interactions become tiring because emotional buffering capacity is narrowed. Physical activity feels heavier because baseline activation and recovery debt have increased operating cost underneath movement itself.

Fatigue then emerges not as emotional fragility, but as accumulated regulation burden.

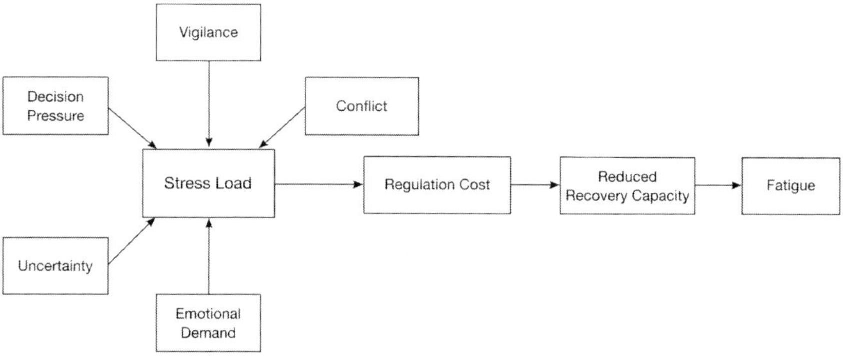


**[Figure 11: Stress Load and Regulation Cost]**

The relationship represented here clarifies why prolonged stress frequently produces exhaustion even without obvious physical overexertion. Sustained vigilance, uncertainty, emotional demand, adaptation pressure, and continuous nervous system activation progressively increase the energetic cost required to maintain ordinary stability. The body reallocates resources toward coordination, prediction, regulation, and adaptation across time. As regulation cost rises, less net usable capacity remains available for concentration, emotional resilience, physical effort, and sustained output.

This framework changes how stress-related fatigue is interpreted. The body is not simply reacting emotionally. It is managing allocation under prolonged demand. Vigilance itself is metabolically expensive. Adaptation consumes resources. Uncertainty increases regulatory burden because the nervous system struggles to fully settle into restoration while potential disruption remains unresolved.

This is why visible inactivity does not necessarily indicate low load. A person can be physiologically exhausted while appearing outwardly still. The nervous system may remain continuously active underneath the absence of visible movement.

Stress also narrows transition flexibility. Moving from activation into recovery becomes more difficult under sustained load. Sleep onset may become harder. Relaxation feels incomplete. Recovery periods lose efficiency. The body struggles to fully shift states because activation has become partially normalized internally.

Fatigue then accumulates because the system never fully exits vigilance long enough to rebuild capacity proportionately.

This pattern frequently creates a sense of being simultaneously tired and activated. The person feels depleted but unable to fully settle. Exhausted but restless. Sleepy but not deeply restored. The body remains trapped between demand and recovery without fully stabilizing inside either condition.

The resulting fatigue is often interpreted psychologically because the symptoms appear emotional or behavioral on the surface. Irritability rises. Motivation fluctuates. Concentration shortens. Tolerance narrows. Avoidance increases. Physiologically, however, the underlying issue may be escalating regulation cost rather than moral weakness or insufficient effort.

The body becomes progressively more expensive to stabilize under sustained stress exposure.

Importantly, the goal is not the elimination of all stress from human life. Stress responses are adaptive. Human beings are built to handle challenge, uncertainty, concentrated effort, emotional intensity, and periods of increased demand. Problems emerge primarily when restoration repeatedly fails to keep pace with the ongoing cost of adaptation across time.

Stable systems are not systems without stress. They are systems where stress activation remains sufficiently balanced by restoration, flexibility, fuel continuity, sleep-recovery translation, and preserved support capacity.

When that balance deteriorates chronically, fatigue becomes increasingly visible because the body is redirecting growing portions of available resources toward maintaining regulation itself.

The resulting exhaustion often feels diffuse because stress affects multiple systems simultaneously. Sleep quality deteriorates. Emotional resilience narrows. Fuel regulation destabilizes. Recovery debt accumulates. Transition friction increases. Utilization cost rises. Ordinary demands become disproportionately heavy.

Fatigue then emerges not from one isolated failure, but from accumulated coordination expense distributed across the entire system.

This interpretation removes much of the shame commonly attached to stress-related exhaustion. The body is not failing because it lacks character. It is carrying sustained adaptation demand across time. The fatigue signal reflects rising physiological allocation toward vigilance, regulation, and continuity maintenance under persistent load.

And as stress continues altering fuel coordination and nervous system signaling, another layer of instability becomes increasingly visible underneath the exhaustion itself. Energy continuity often becomes more variable under prolonged activation, with shifts in glucose stability contributing to crashes, fog, irritability, uneven output, and unstable usable function across time.

# Glucose Variability Mechanism

Fatigue does not always arrive gradually. Some forms of exhaustion emerge sharply, almost abruptly, with sudden heaviness, fog, irritability, shakiness, narrowing tolerance, unstable concentration, or an urgent feeling that usable function has collapsed within a relatively short period of time. These experiences often feel different from slower forms of accumulated fatigue. The body may appear functional one hour and disproportionately strained the next. Output becomes unstable rather than simply low.

One important contributor to this pattern is glucose variability.

Glucose variability is not the sole explanation for fatigue, nor should fatigue be reduced simplistically to blood sugar alone. Human exhaustion remains shaped by recovery debt, stress load, sleep disruption, utilization cost, nervous system strain, immune demand, transition friction, and broader load-capacity mismatch across time. Glucose variability matters because it can amplify fatigue patterns by disrupting energy continuity and increasing regulation cost underneath ordinary function.

The Glucose Variability Mechanism describes this directly: fatigue can be amplified when glucose availability rises, falls, or fluctuates in ways that disrupt energy continuity and increase regulation cost.

This distinction matters because fatigue linked to unstable glucose availability often feels qualitatively different from slower forms of depletion. General under-recovery may feel dense, heavy, and persistent. Glucose instability frequently feels sharper, more sudden, more irritable, more foggy, and more unstable. Concentration narrows abruptly.

Emotional tolerance shortens. Physical heaviness appears quickly. Motivation becomes erratic. Cognitive continuity weakens. The body shifts rapidly from relatively functional output into reduced usable function.

The experience often feels urgent because fuel continuity itself has become unstable.

Glucose functions as one of the body's most visible fuel signals. Blood sugar levels continuously reflect the interaction among intake, insulin signaling, liver glucose release, stress state, activity demand, recovery condition, and ongoing metabolic coordination. Stable energy continuity depends partly on the body's ability to maintain sufficiently coordinated glucose availability across changing conditions.

This does not mean glucose must remain perfectly flat or unchanging. Human physiology naturally involves fluctuation. Meals increase availability. Activity changes demand. Fasting states alter fuel sourcing. Stress shifts allocation priorities. The issue is not fluctuation itself. The issue is whether variability becomes large enough, rapid enough, or poorly coordinated enough that usable function becomes unstable.

Under relatively stable conditions, glucose availability moves dynamically without producing excessive disruption. Energy continuity remains reasonably preserved across ordinary life. Concentration stays accessible. Emotional regulation remains manageable. Physical function remains relatively smooth.

Under unstable conditions, however, glucose availability may rise and fall in ways that amplify fatigue sharply.

The body then spends increasing amounts of effort preserving continuity underneath fluctuating fuel conditions.

This instability can emerge through several overlapping pathways. Delayed meals may create widening gaps between current demand and available fuel accessibility. Stress activation may increase glucose release temporarily while simultaneously destabilizing longer-term regulation.

Sleep disruption may impair insulin signaling coordination and increase variability across the following day. Recovery debt may narrow the system's ability to buffer energetic fluctuation smoothly. High cognitive demand or emotional strain may increase energetic requirements while regulation remains unstable underneath.

The result is often a fatigue pattern defined by inconsistency rather than simple depletion.

Crashes are one of the clearest examples. A crash is not merely feeling tired. It often involves sudden narrowing of usable function accompanied by fog, shakiness, irritability, urgency, emotional volatility, heaviness, reduced tolerance, or abrupt decline in concentration. The body shifts quickly into a state where sustaining ordinary output becomes disproportionately difficult.

These experiences frequently reflect instability in glucose continuity relative to current demand.

Insulin signaling plays a central role in this coordination process because insulin helps regulate fuel movement, storage, access, and distribution across tissues. Insulin is not a villain or enemy signal. It is part of the body's coordination architecture. The system continuously adjusts fuel allocation according to current energetic conditions.

Under stable conditions, this coordination preserves relatively smooth continuity between incoming fuel, stored reserves, tissue uptake, and ongoing demand. Under strained conditions, timing and regulation may become less synchronized. Glucose availability may rise rapidly, decline sharply, or fail to remain sufficiently continuous relative to the energetic demands being placed on the system.

The resulting fatigue often feels metabolically abrupt because fuel accessibility itself has become unstable.

This instability is influenced by more than intake alone. Glucose availability depends partly on meal timing, but also on liver glucose release, stress signaling, nervous system activation, sleep quality, recovery state, activity demand, hormonal coordination, and broader metabolic flexibility. A person may therefore experience unstable energy continuity even without dramatic changes in food intake itself.

Stress load is especially important here because prolonged activation alters glucose regulation continuously. Acute stress can temporarily increase glucose availability to support immediate demand. Cortisol and broader stress signaling help mobilize fuel under perceived threat or pressure. In the short term, this process is adaptive. The body increases energetic accessibility in order to preserve function during challenge.

Under sustained stress exposure, however, this repeated activation often destabilizes continuity across time.

Glucose availability becomes more reactive. Crashes become sharper. Irritability increases. Concentration becomes less stable. Emotional tolerance narrows more quickly. The body spends increasing amounts of effort attempting to coordinate fuel continuity underneath ongoing activation.

This interaction explains why stress-related fatigue often includes periods of temporary alertness followed by abrupt exhaustion afterward. Activation temporarily increases usable function while simultaneously increasing regulation cost and destabilizing longer-term continuity.

The resulting fatigue is not merely emotional. It is energetic instability occurring within a stressed system.

Poor sleep amplifies these patterns substantially because sleep quality influences glucose regulation across the following day. Sleep disruption alters insulin signaling coordination, stress responsiveness, appetite regulation, nervous system stability, and broader metabolic timing. The body then becomes less able to buffer ordinary fluctuations smoothly.

Glucose variability often becomes more noticeable under these conditions because the system possesses less reserve available for adaptation.

Recovery debt compounds this instability further. A well-rested system generally tolerates ordinary energetic fluctuation more smoothly because reserve capacity remains broader. Under-recovered systems possess narrower stability margins. Small disruptions therefore produce larger experiential consequences. Delayed meals feel more destabilizing. Stress responses become sharper. Crashes appear more quickly. Emotional resilience declines faster.

The body becomes less flexible in its ability to maintain energy continuity under changing conditions.

Importantly, this mechanism should not become glucose panic or dietary moralization. Human physiology naturally involves changing glucose levels across feeding, fasting, activity, recovery, and stress states. The existence of fluctuation is not inherently pathological. The issue is interpretive. Certain patterns of instability can amplify fatigue experiences by increasing regulation cost and disrupting usable continuity.

The goal here is explanation rather than prescription.

This distinction matters because many discussions around glucose become overly rigid, fearful, or reductionistic. Fatigue cannot be explained entirely through carbohydrates, insulin, meal timing, or singular dietary rules. Glucose variability is one layer inside a much broader system involving stress load, sleep-recovery translation, fuel access, nervous system regulation, recovery debt, immune strain, and overall support capacity.

The body is not merely responding to food. It is coordinating energy continuity across changing conditions.

This coordination becomes especially difficult under cumulative strain. Stress load, poor sleep, emotional burden, transition friction, and rising utilization cost all increase the energetic expense required to maintain stable function. The body then becomes more sensitive to instability because the margin for fluctuation narrows progressively.

Under these conditions, glucose swings often feel more dramatic because the system has fewer reserves available to buffer disruption smoothly.

A person may therefore tolerate ordinary variability relatively well under stable conditions while experiencing pronounced crashes under periods of high stress or poor recovery. The same energetic fluctuation interacts differently with different system states.

The body responds contextually rather than mechanically.

This also explains why glucose-related fatigue often appears alongside irritability, shakiness, narrowed patience, reduced emotional tolerance, or cognitive fog rather than only simple tiredness. The nervous system depends partly on stable fuel continuity. When availability becomes unstable, broader regulation quality often becomes unstable alongside it.

The resulting fatigue therefore feels multidimensional. Emotional resilience weakens. Cognitive clarity fades. Physical heaviness rises. Concentration fragments. Motivation becomes inconsistent. The body experiences not only reduced energy, but reduced continuity of usable function itself.

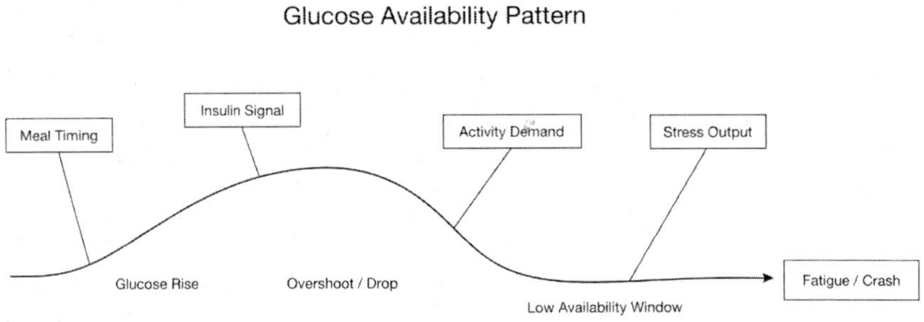


**[Figure 12: Glucose Variability and Fatigue]**

The sequence represented here clarifies why unstable glucose availability can amplify fatigue patterns so sharply. Glucose rises in response to intake, stress output, or changing energetic conditions. Under certain strained circumstances, the regulation response overshoots or availability drops too quickly relative to current demand. A low-availability window emerges where usable fuel continuity narrows abruptly. The result is the fatigue or crash pattern many people experience as fog, irritability, shakiness, heaviness, reduced tolerance, or sudden loss of usable function. Meal timing, insulin coordination, activity demand, and stress signaling all influence how smoothly these transitions occur.

This framework helps explain why some fatigue feels unstable rather than continuously flat. Energy appears accessible temporarily before collapsing abruptly afterward. Concentration fluctuates unpredictably. Motivation rises and falls sharply. Emotional tolerance narrows suddenly during periods of reduced availability.

The issue is often not total absence of fuel, but instability in continuity and coordination.

This understanding also restores proportion to the interpretation of glucose itself. Blood sugar variability matters because the body depends partly on stable fuel continuity in order to preserve smooth function across time. Yet glucose remains one mechanism within a larger fatigue system rather than the universal explanation for all exhaustion.

The body cannot be reduced to a single fuel variable.

Stress load still matters. Recovery debt still matters. Sleep-recovery translation still matters. Utilization cost still matters. Immune strain, nervous system activation, emotional demand, and broader load-capacity mismatch all remain deeply relevant. Glucose variability amplifies fatigue partly because unstable fuel continuity increases regulation expense inside systems already carrying other forms of strain.

This amplification effect explains why crashes often feel disproportionately disruptive during periods of stress or under-recovery.

The body is already operating with narrowed reserve. Glucose instability then further destabilizes continuity, making fatigue feel sharper and more difficult to stabilize.

The resulting experience is often interpreted emotionally or morally because the shifts feel abrupt and difficult to control consciously. A person may feel functional, motivated, and emotionally stable before suddenly becoming irritable, foggy, shaky, exhausted, or unable to sustain ordinary concentration.

Physiologically, the system may simply be struggling to maintain coordinated fuel continuity under strained conditions.

This interpretation changes the relationship between fatigue and glucose entirely. The body is not failing morally because energy continuity became unstable. Fatigue in these moments frequently reflects rising regulation cost underneath fluctuating fuel availability.

The goal is therefore not fear, perfection, or rigid control. The goal is interpretive clarity.

Glucose variability does not explain all fatigue, but unstable glucose availability can sharpen fatigue into crashes, fog, irritability, reduced tolerance, and unstable output when energy continuity becomes difficult to maintain smoothly across time.

And as energetic continuity becomes increasingly difficult to coordinate under broader strain, another layer of fatigue begins emerging underneath fuel instability itself. The body also depends on stable fluid balance and electrolyte signaling in order to maintain communication, circulation, muscular coordination, and usable function across systems.

## Electrolyte Signal Mechanism

Fatigue does not always feel sharp, unstable, or crash-like. Some forms of exhaustion feel heavier, flatter, weaker, slower, more diffuse, or strangely difficult to interpret clearly. The body may not feel abruptly depleted so much as broadly diminished. Muscular coordination feels less stable. Physical movement becomes effortful without obvious explanation. Cognitive clarity softens. Tolerance narrows. The system feels less responsive overall, as though communication itself has become less precise.

One important contributor to this pattern is electrolyte signal integrity.

Electrolytes are often discussed almost exclusively through hydration culture, supplementation trends, or performance language, but fatigue reveals a broader systems role. Sodium, potassium, magnesium, and fluid balance are not merely accessories to hydration. They participate continuously in signaling quality, fluid distribution, muscular coordination, circulation, and nervous system regulation across the body.

The Electrolyte Signal Mechanism describes this directly: fatigue can become heavier, flatter, weaker, or more diffuse when fluid balance and electrolyte signaling reduce the body's ability to coordinate usable function.

This distinction matters because the body depends not only on fuel availability, but also on communication quality. Energy alone does not produce stable function automatically. Signals must move appropriately. Muscles must contract efficiently. Circulation must adapt continuously.

Nerve signaling must remain coordinated. Fluid distribution must remain sufficiently stable across changing conditions.

When these coordination processes become strained, fatigue often changes character.

The exhaustion may feel less like a dramatic crash and more like broad instability in function itself. Physical heaviness increases. Movement feels less efficient. Tolerance declines. Cognitive sharpness softens. The body feels flat rather than energized, diffuse rather than focused.

This fatigue often feels difficult to interpret because the system's signaling quality itself has become less stable.

Electrolytes participate in this coordination continuously. Sodium helps regulate fluid balance and signaling gradients. Potassium contributes to muscular and nerve communication. Magnesium participates across numerous coordination and regulatory processes involving muscular function, signaling stability, and energetic regulation. Fluid balance itself influences circulation, pressure relationships, tissue communication, and broader system continuity.

These elements operate together as part of signal integrity architecture rather than as isolated inputs.

Under relatively stable conditions, signaling quality remains coordinated enough that ordinary function feels reasonably smooth. Muscles respond proportionately. Circulation adjusts appropriately. Cognitive continuity remains stable. Physical effort matches demand relatively predictably.

Under strained conditions, however, fluid distribution and signaling quality may become less stable. The body then spends increasing effort attempting to preserve coordination underneath impaired communication conditions.

The resulting fatigue frequently feels physically heavy because muscular efficiency itself becomes less smooth. The nervous system must work harder to maintain coordination. Circulation becomes less adaptive.

Tolerance narrows because ordinary demands consume more effort than expected.

This experience differs from glucose crashes in important ways. Glucose variability often produces abrupt instability, urgency, irritability, shakiness, or sudden narrowing of usable function. Electrolyte-related strain often feels flatter, heavier, slower, weaker, or more diffuse. The system does not necessarily feel abruptly depleted so much as broadly less coordinated.

The body feels harder to operate.

This distinction also separates electrolyte signal disruption from recovery debt. Recovery debt frequently feels dense and cumulative, as though reserve capacity has narrowed progressively across time. Electrolyte instability often feels more immediate and coordination-oriented. Muscles feel less responsive. Physical tolerance drops unexpectedly. Fog increases. Movement becomes disproportionately effortful. Circulation feels less adaptive. The body feels less structurally stable under ordinary demand.

The signaling layer underneath usable function has become strained.

Fluid balance is central to this process because communication quality depends partly on stable distribution relationships throughout the body. Circulation, muscular contraction, nerve signaling, tissue responsiveness, and energetic continuity all rely on coordinated fluid movement and signaling gradients across systems.

The body therefore experiences fluid instability not simply as thirst, but often as altered functional continuity.

This helps explain why fatigue associated with fluid and electrolyte instability can feel difficult to describe clearly. A person may not feel dramatically sleepy or emotionally exhausted. Instead, the body feels weak, flat, heavy, disconnected, or strangely inefficient. The system appears less responsive overall.

Because the fatigue lacks a single dramatic feature, people often dismiss or misinterpret it.

Stress load can contribute substantially to this instability because stress alters fluid distribution, signaling demand, and regulatory burden continuously. Nervous system activation changes circulation patterns, muscular tension, and energetic allocation. Persistent stress also increases broader regulation cost, making the system more vulnerable to coordination instability underneath ongoing demand.

The resulting fatigue frequently combines heaviness with reduced tolerance. Ordinary exertion becomes disproportionately effortful. Recovery slows. Physical steadiness decreases. Cognitive continuity weakens.

The body is attempting to maintain coordination under rising signaling strain.

Heat and sweating influence this process because fluid balance shifts dynamically under thermal and exertional demand. Human physiology is adaptive and capable of managing these transitions under many conditions, but prolonged strain, recovery debt, inadequate restoration, or ongoing stress may narrow the stability margin available for smooth adjustment.

The resulting fatigue often reflects coordination strain rather than simple absence of energy.

Illness can create similar patterns because immune strain alters fluid balance, circulation, signaling demand, and broader regulation simultaneously. The body reallocates resources toward repair, defense, and continuity maintenance. Electrolyte and fluid instability may then contribute to diffuse exhaustion, muscular heaviness, weakness, or reduced functional tolerance.

Again, the issue is not merely hydration in the simplistic sense. The issue is coordination quality across systems.

Poor sleep amplifies these effects because sleep disruption interferes with restoration broadly. Nervous system downshifting becomes incomplete. Recovery debt accumulates. Stress signaling remains elevated. Fuel continuity becomes less stable. The body therefore enters subsequent days with narrower reserve available for maintaining signaling integrity smoothly under ordinary demand.

The resulting fatigue often feels compounded. Heaviness, fog, reduced tolerance, unstable concentration, muscular strain, and lowered resilience overlap simultaneously because multiple coordination systems are carrying unresolved burden together.

Fasting and broader energetic transitions can also influence electrolyte strain because shifting fuel states alter fluid movement and signaling relationships dynamically. This does not make fasting inherently harmful or beneficial. Human physiology continuously adapts across feeding and fasting conditions. The important point is interpretive. Under certain strained circumstances, energetic transitions may interact with fluid balance and signaling continuity in ways that amplify fatigue.

The resulting exhaustion often reflects coordination instability rather than singular fuel absence.

Importantly, this mechanism should not become supplement culture or dosing language. Electrolyte signal integrity cannot be reduced simplistically to consuming more sodium, potassium, magnesium, or fluids. Human physiology regulates these relationships dynamically through interacting systems involving stress state, sleep quality, activity demand, hormonal coordination, recovery status, circulation, kidney regulation, energetic continuity, and broader system stability.

The goal here is interpretation rather than correction protocols.

This distinction matters because many conversations about electrolytes drift quickly into rigid behavioral rules. The body is more dynamic than isolated intake targets. Fatigue linked to signaling instability reflects broader coordination strain rather than merely the absence of one nutrient in isolation.

Electrolyte integrity therefore belongs inside a systems framework rather than inside simplistic optimization culture.

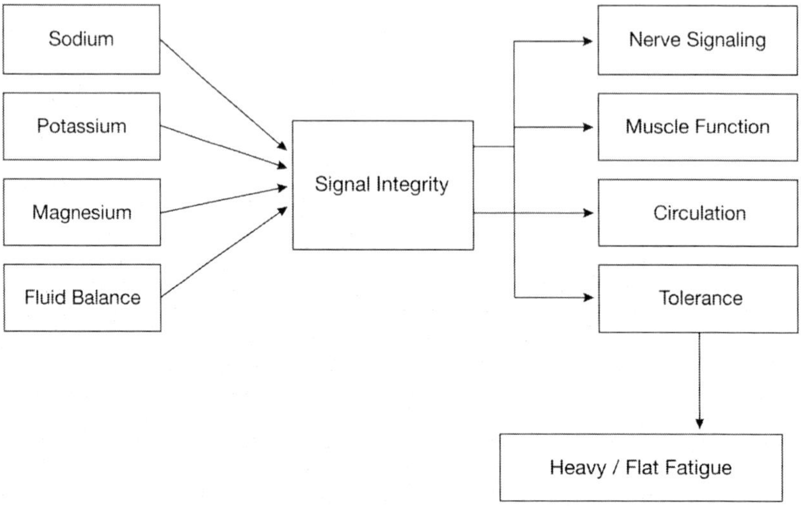


**[Figure 13: Electrolyte Signal Integrity]**

The relationship represented here clarifies why electrolyte and fluid instability can alter fatigue quality so significantly. Sodium, potassium, magnesium, and fluid balance contribute collectively to signal integrity across the body. Signaling quality then influences nerve communication, muscular function, circulation, and overall tolerance for demand. When coordination becomes unstable, fatigue often shifts toward heaviness, flatness, weakness, fog, or diffuse reduction in usable function. The issue is not simply energy supply alone, but the body's ability to coordinate communication efficiently enough to sustain stable output.

This framework changes how certain forms of exhaustion are interpreted. The body is not necessarily lacking motivation or refusing effort. Signaling quality itself may be strained. The system is attempting to maintain coordinated function while fluid balance, muscular communication, circulation, and nervous system regulation require increasing effort to stabilize.

The resulting fatigue therefore feels broader and less sharply defined than many other fatigue patterns.

This also explains why ordinary tasks can feel unusually effortful under electrolyte strain. Muscular coordination becomes less efficient. Circulatory adjustment becomes less smooth. Nervous system signaling requires greater regulation effort. Tolerance narrows because maintaining stable output consumes disproportionate capacity underneath seemingly simple activity.

The body becomes more expensive to coordinate.

Importantly, electrolyte signal integrity is only one layer within a much larger fatigue system. Recovery debt, stress load, glucose variability, sleep-recovery translation, utilization cost, immune strain, and broader load-capacity mismatch all remain deeply relevant. Electrolyte disruption amplifies fatigue partly because unstable communication quality makes every other regulatory process more difficult to sustain smoothly.

The body depends on coordination across systems rather than isolated energy alone.

This understanding also removes some of the confusion surrounding diffuse exhaustion. A person may feel physically weak, mentally flat, emotionally narrowed, and generally unstable without identifying one obvious cause. Physiologically, signaling quality itself may be contributing to the experience. The system feels difficult to stabilize because communication efficiency has become less reliable under strain.

The resulting fatigue is often harder to interpret precisely because it lacks the dramatic sharpness of glucose crashes or the obvious cumulative heaviness of prolonged recovery debt. Instead, the body simply feels less coherent in its ability to sustain smooth function across ordinary demands.

This diffuse quality often causes people to underestimate the physiological significance of what they are experiencing. The fatigue feels vague, yet the reduction in usable function can still be substantial.

The important shift is interpretive clarity. Electrolytes are not merely hydration accessories or performance tools. They participate continuously in signal integrity, fluid coordination, muscular responsiveness, circulation, and nervous system regulation. When those coordination processes become unstable, fatigue often becomes heavier, flatter, weaker, foggier, or harder to interpret clearly.

The body is not simply low on energy. The signaling architecture supporting usable function may itself be strained.

And when signaling instability overlaps with stress load, recovery debt, glucose variability, and ongoing adaptation pressure, another pattern often begins emerging underneath visible function itself. Fatigue does not always immediately stop performance. Caffeine, urgency, adrenaline, habit, obligation, and continuous activation can temporarily preserve output even while the underlying physiological debt continues rising underneath the appearance of normal function.

# Compensation Mechanism

Fatigue does not always reduce visible function immediately. Human physiology possesses multiple ways of preserving output temporarily even while underlying strain continues accumulating underneath. A person may continue working, caregiving, concentrating, performing socially, training, responding to deadlines, or maintaining routines while simultaneously carrying substantial recovery debt, rising regulation cost, unstable fuel continuity, nervous system strain, and narrowing support capacity.

The visible continuation of function often creates the impression that the system remains adequately restored. Physiologically, however, functioning and recovering are not identical conditions.

This distinction becomes especially important when fatigue is partially masked through compensation.

The Compensation Mechanism describes this directly: fatigue can be masked when temporary output support preserves visible function while underlying strain, recovery debt, or regulation cost continues rising.

Compensation is not inherently pathological or irrational. Human physiology depends on adaptive compensation continuously. Acute stress signaling preserves performance during emergencies. Adrenal activation increases vigilance under immediate demand. Habit and routine reduce cognitive burden by automating repeated actions. Social obligation maintains continuity during difficult periods. Urgency narrows attention toward immediate priorities. Caffeine increases alertness temporarily.

Identity and responsibility help sustain effort during circumstances where withdrawal from demand is not immediately possible.

These processes can be highly adaptive in the short term.

The problem emerges when compensation becomes confused with restoration itself.

Visible output may continue while the underlying conditions required for stable long-term function continue deteriorating quietly underneath. Recovery debt still accumulates. Stress activation remains elevated. Sleep-recovery translation remains incomplete. Fuel instability persists. Nervous system strain continues rising. Utilization cost remains elevated.

The system therefore appears externally functional while internally becoming progressively more expensive to sustain.

This distinction explains why many people do not fully recognize fatigue until compensation begins failing. During the compensatory phase, the body preserves continuity through increasing activation and regulation effort. Responsibilities continue being met. Deadlines are handled. Work remains possible. Social obligations continue. The person may even appear highly productive or outwardly energetic.

Underneath that preserved output, however, the body may be reallocating increasing amounts of resources simply to maintain ordinary function.

Compensation therefore often delays visibility rather than eliminating strain.

Caffeine is one of the clearest examples because it can temporarily increase alertness and reduce the immediate perception of fatigue. This effect is not inherently harmful or deceptive. The body uses multiple forms of activation support naturally. The important distinction is interpretive. Increased alertness does not automatically mean restored capacity.

A person may feel temporarily more functional while the underlying recovery debt remains unresolved.

This distinction matters because many fatigue patterns become difficult to interpret precisely when compensation is effective. The individual sees continued output and assumes the system must therefore be adequately restored. Physiologically, however, the body may simply be maintaining function through increasing activation cost.

The system continues operating, but at greater expense.

Urgency produces similar effects. During periods of immediate pressure, human physiology often narrows focus toward task completion and survival continuity. Fatigue signals may become partially suppressed because the body prioritizes immediate adaptation over restorative awareness. Concentration sharpens temporarily. Energy feels temporarily more accessible. Emotional buffering narrows toward functional necessity.

Once the urgent period ends, the accumulated fatigue frequently becomes much more visible.

This delayed exhaustion is not sudden weakness appearing randomly afterward. It is often the previously masked cost of maintaining output under sustained activation.

Adrenaline functions similarly. Acute activation can temporarily increase available output substantially. The body reallocates resources toward immediate action, vigilance, and performance continuity. Under short-term conditions, this process is highly adaptive. Human beings are built to function under temporary periods of concentrated demand.

When activation becomes prolonged, however, the energetic cost rises steadily underneath the preserved output.

The body begins spending increasing resources maintaining the activated state itself. Sleep quality declines. Recovery efficiency weakens. Emotional resilience narrows. Fuel continuity destabilizes. Ordinary tasks begin consuming more effort than expected.

Compensation preserves visible continuity while reducing future stability margin underneath.

Habit and routine also operate as compensation layers because repeated behavior decreases decision burden and preserves continuity even under reduced capacity. A person may continue fulfilling responsibilities largely through momentum and familiarity despite significant underlying fatigue. This is not evidence that fatigue is absent. It often reflects the body conserving function by reducing the energetic cost of behavioral initiation and adaptation.

Routine allows visible performance to continue even while reserve capacity narrows.

Social pressure and obligation can intensify this process further. Human beings frequently continue functioning under strain because others depend on them, because expectations remain active, because roles must be maintained, or because stopping feels impossible within current circumstances. Caregiving, parenting, professional obligations, financial pressure, and relational responsibilities all create strong continuity demands that preserve output despite exhaustion.

The body therefore continues reallocating resources toward functioning even when restoration remains incomplete.

Importantly, this should not be framed morally either positively or negatively. Compensation is neither proof of strength nor evidence of dysfunction automatically. It is an adaptive regulatory strategy. The body attempts to preserve continuity under difficult conditions using the tools available to it.

The key issue is that compensation changes visibility more than it changes underlying strain itself.

This explains why some individuals appear highly functional externally while privately carrying profound exhaustion. Visible output alone does not reliably measure restored capacity. A person may continue performing effectively through increasing activation, pressure, obligation, and compensatory regulation while simultaneously becoming progressively more unstable underneath.

The body can preserve performance surprisingly long before obvious collapse occurs.

This preservation often creates interpretive confusion because people assume fatigue should immediately reduce visible function proportionately. Physiologically, the system frequently compensates first. Only later does the accumulated cost become too large to continue masking effectively.

This delayed recognition is one reason fatigue often feels sudden even when the underlying strain accumulated gradually.

The "crash" appears abrupt because compensation had previously concealed the narrowing stability margin underneath.

Recovery debt plays a major role here because compensation frequently allows under-recovery to continue accumulating invisibly across time. The person continues functioning through activation, obligation, caffeine, routine, and urgency while restoration repeatedly falls short of demand. Because visible output remains intact, the underlying debt remains difficult to recognize clearly.

The body therefore carries unresolved strain forward silently underneath ongoing productivity.

Stress load compounds this process because sustained activation itself increases regulation cost continuously. The body spends more energy maintaining vigilance, emotional buffering, cognitive continuity, and adaptation while simultaneously attempting to preserve ordinary function. Compensation layers then further extend output despite rising internal expense.

Eventually the operating cost becomes difficult to sustain.

This explains why delayed crashes often occur after prolonged periods of apparently successful functioning. The body had been compensating successfully enough to preserve visible continuity temporarily. Once activation decreases, deadlines end, obligations loosen, or adrenaline subsides, the accumulated strain becomes harder to continue suppressing.

The resulting exhaustion often feels disproportionate because the visible workload may have already decreased substantially by the time the crash occurs.

Physiologically, the crash frequently reflects accumulated regulation cost finally becoming visible rather than sudden collapse emerging from nowhere.

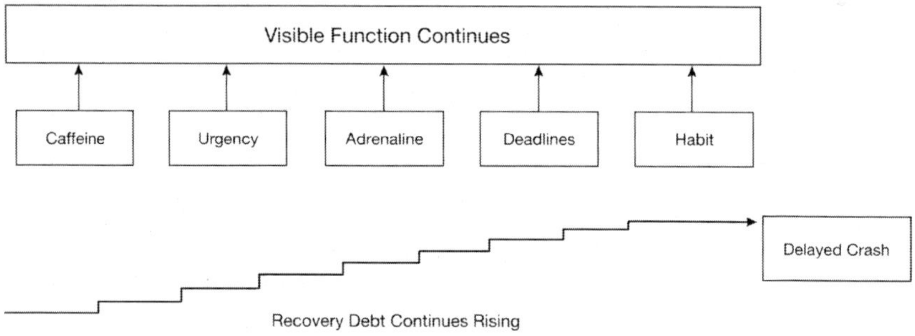


**[Figure 14: Compensation Mask]**

The relationship represented here clarifies why compensation frequently obscures fatigue interpretation. Visible function continues through temporary support layers such as caffeine, urgency, adrenaline, deadlines, and habit. Outwardly, the system appears productive and stable. Underneath that preserved output, however, recovery debt and regulation cost continue rising across time. Eventually the stability margin narrows enough that delayed fatigue becomes more visible once compensation weakens or activation decreases.

This framework changes how functioning under strain is interpreted. Continued output does not automatically prove restored capacity. The body may simply be preserving continuity through increasing compensatory effort.

The distinction between functioning and recovering becomes especially important here. Human beings can often function under substantial strain temporarily. Recovery, however, requires actual rebuilding of support capacity rather than merely preservation of visible output.

The body therefore may continue producing performance while simultaneously becoming less restored underneath.

This also explains why some people feel unexpectedly exhausted during periods that appear externally calmer. Once activation decreases, the body no longer suppresses fatigue signals with the same intensity. The unresolved debt becomes easier to feel. The person may assume they are becoming weaker because fatigue appeared after the stressful period rather than during it.

Physiologically, compensation had simply delayed visibility.

This delayed visibility often creates shame because modern culture frequently rewards visible performance without recognizing the underlying physiological cost required to sustain it. A person may continue meeting obligations while quietly carrying substantial nervous system strain, unstable recovery, glucose variability, emotional exhaustion, and rising utilization cost underneath.

The body eventually reveals the accumulated expense regardless of how successfully output was temporarily preserved.

Importantly, compensation itself should not be demonized. Temporary output support is often necessary. Human life contains periods where adaptation, responsibility, and sustained functioning are unavoidable. The body's ability to preserve continuity under demand is part of its adaptive intelligence.

The issue is not that compensation exists. The issue is whether compensation becomes mistaken for restoration itself.

When visible functioning is interpreted as proof of recovered capacity, underlying strain may continue accumulating unnoticed. Recovery debt deepens. Stress activation persists. Sleep quality deteriorates. Fuel continuity destabilizes. Signal integrity weakens. The stability margin narrows progressively underneath ongoing output preservation.

Fatigue then becomes harder to interpret because the person appears functional right up until the system can no longer maintain compensation comfortably.

This understanding changes the meaning of delayed exhaustion entirely. The crash after prolonged demand is not necessarily evidence of sudden weakness, lack of resilience, or personal failure. It is often accumulated cost finally becoming visible once the compensatory layer can no longer fully conceal the underlying strain.

The body had been spending resources maintaining continuity all along.

Fatigue therefore may remain partially hidden even while the system becomes progressively more expensive to stabilize underneath ordinary function. Compensation preserves output temporarily, but the underlying physiological debt continues accumulating beneath the appearance of continuity.

And eventually, when the body determines that preserving current output threatens broader stability too severely, another regulatory shift often occurs. Rather than merely signaling fatigue while maintaining performance, the system may begin actively reducing available function itself through protective downshifting.

## Downshift Mechanism

Fatigue does not always appear as complete collapse. More often, the body reduces access to output gradually before deeper instability occurs. Motivation narrows. Movement slows. Concentration shortens. Emotional tolerance decreases. Social interaction becomes more effortful. Decision-making feels disproportionately heavy. Task initiation weakens. Activities that once felt neutral begin requiring unusual effort simply to begin and sustain.

These changes are frequently interpreted psychologically. A person may conclude they have become lazy, weak, undisciplined, emotionally fragile, unmotivated, or unwilling to exert effort. The visible reduction in drive appears voluntary because the body is still technically capable of some degree of function.

Physiologically, however, the system may be actively reducing accessible output in order to preserve stability under constrained conditions.

This reduction is downshift.

The Downshift Mechanism describes this directly: fatigue can appear when the body reduces available output in order to protect stability under conditions of rising strain, narrowed capacity, or excessive regulation cost.

This distinction matters because fatigue is often expected to remain purely informational. Earlier fatigue signals may appear as heaviness, crashes, fog, reduced continuity, unstable tolerance, or growing effort cost while visible function remains relatively intact. Downshift represents a deeper regulatory shift. The body begins not only signaling strain, but limiting output itself.

The reduction is protective rather than punitive.

Human physiology does not wait for catastrophic collapse before altering behavior. The body continuously adjusts access to exertion, focus, emotional engagement, social tolerance, and sustained activity according to current support capacity. When strain rises high enough relative to available restoration and regulation reserve, the system often narrows output intentionally in order to reduce additional destabilization.

This narrowing frequently feels frustrating because the person's intentions may remain unchanged while the body's willingness to sustain output declines sharply.

The distinction between intention and accessible function becomes especially visible here. A person may genuinely want to concentrate, socialize, exercise, work, respond emotionally, or complete responsibilities while simultaneously experiencing profound resistance to initiating and sustaining those actions.

The issue is not necessarily absence of desire. The system may simply be restricting output availability underneath conscious intention.

This helps explain why downshift is so commonly misread as motivational failure. The person often appears externally capable of action while internally experiencing strong reduction in accessible drive and tolerance. Because no obvious structural injury is visible, the reduction is interpreted morally rather than physiologically.

The body is frequently responding to cumulative strain rather than to weakness of character.

Compensation and downshift represent opposite regulatory directions. Compensation preserves visible output temporarily despite rising strain. Downshift reduces visible output because preserving prior levels has become too expensive relative to available support capacity.

Compensation says: maintain continuity despite cost.

Downshift says: reduce cost to preserve continuity.

This distinction is important because many fatigue patterns move through both phases sequentially. The body first preserves function through activation, urgency, caffeine, stress signaling, habit, obligation, and narrowed attention. Over time, recovery debt accumulates, regulation cost rises, fuel continuity destabilizes, sleep-recovery translation weakens, and nervous system strain increases.

Eventually the compensatory layer becomes increasingly difficult to sustain.

The body then begins reducing accessible output before deeper disruption occurs.

This reduction may appear as lower motivation, slower movement, reduced emotional engagement, narrowed social tolerance, shortened concentration, decreased willingness to initiate tasks, or increased resistance toward effort generally. The person may still technically function, but ordinary actions feel metabolically expensive in ways that are difficult to override sustainably.

The body begins enforcing boundaries through reduced accessibility itself.

Recovery debt strongly contributes to this process because unresolved restoration progressively narrows reserve capacity across time. A well-rested system generally tolerates ordinary demands flexibly. An under-recovered system must allocate resources more carefully because the stability margin has already been reduced.

The body therefore becomes more selective about where output remains accessible.

Stress load amplifies downshift because prolonged vigilance and activation increase operating cost continuously. Emotional buffering, cognitive continuity, fuel regulation, muscular tension, and nervous system coordination all require increasing resources under sustained strain.

The system eventually recognizes that maintaining prior output levels would continue widening the restoration gap.

Downshift then functions partly as boundary enforcement against further destabilization.

This enforcement often appears psychologically before it appears physically. A person may notice shrinking patience, lower emotional bandwidth, reduced willingness to engage socially, decreased tolerance for noise or interruption, increased avoidance of cognitively expensive tasks, or unusual resistance toward obligations that previously felt manageable.

These experiences are frequently interpreted as personality changes or attitude problems.

Physiologically, the system may be reducing discretionary output because available support capacity has narrowed too far to sustain previous levels comfortably.

Utilization cost contributes heavily here as well. Earlier chapters established that energy production alone does not determine usable function. The body may possess fuel while still spending increasing amounts of energy maintaining regulation itself. Stress signaling, poor sleep, immune strain, glucose instability, fluid imbalance, and ongoing adaptation all increase the operating expense required to sustain ordinary activity.

Eventually the body limits output because maintaining prior levels costs too much relative to recoverable capacity.

This protective reduction explains why ordinary tasks begin feeling disproportionately demanding under accumulated strain. The tasks themselves may not have changed substantially. The system carrying them has changed. Attention regulation consumes more energy. Emotional engagement costs more. Decision-making becomes metabolically expensive. Physical movement requires more support. Social interaction demands more buffering capacity.

The body therefore narrows output in order to reduce additional load.

Glucose variability can intensify this process because unstable energy continuity further increases regulation burden underneath ordinary activity. Crashes, fog, irritability, and fluctuating usable function reduce the system's confidence in sustaining prolonged output smoothly. The body responds partly by reducing willingness to engage in energetically expensive tasks unless absolutely necessary.

The resulting reduction often feels like loss of drive, but the deeper issue is reduced confidence in available continuity.

Electrolyte and fluid instability can contribute similarly because signaling quality affects coordination broadly. When muscular responsiveness, circulation, and nervous system signaling become less stable, the body experiences ordinary exertion as increasingly costly. Downshift then reduces activity partly to preserve coordination integrity under strained conditions.

Poor sleep amplifies all of these patterns because restoration quality influences reserve capacity directly. When sleep fails to fully rebuild support capacity, the body begins subsequent days already carrying narrowed tolerance and elevated regulation cost. Downshift becomes more likely because the system possesses less reserve available to absorb ordinary demand comfortably.

The resulting fatigue often feels emotionally confusing because the person remembers previously functioning at higher levels under similar circumstances. The reduction in drive and tolerance therefore feels personal or psychological rather than physiological.

Human physiology, however, adjusts output according to current system state rather than according to past identity.

This distinction removes some of the shame commonly attached to exhaustion. A person experiencing downshift is not necessarily becoming weak, lazy, or unwilling. The body may be reducing access to output because continuing at previous levels would threaten broader stability under current conditions.

The reduction functions partly as preservation.

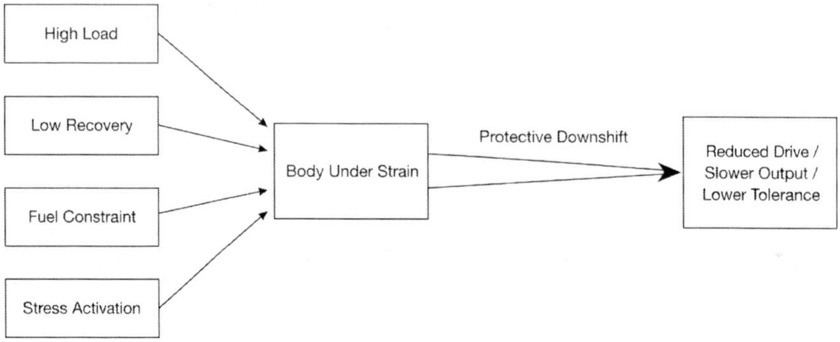


**[Figure 15: Protective Downshift]**

The relationship represented here clarifies why downshift frequently emerges after prolonged strain accumulation. High load, low recovery, fuel constraint, and sustained stress activation all increase regulation cost while narrowing available support capacity. The body under strain then reduces output accessibility through lower drive, slower function, narrowed tolerance, and reduced willingness to sustain exertion. This narrowing is protective rather than punitive. The system is attempting to preserve stability by limiting additional expenditure under constrained conditions.

This framework changes how reduced motivation and lowered output are interpreted. The body is not merely refusing effort irrationally. It may be recalibrating accessibility according to available reserve. Attention, emotional engagement, concentration, social interaction, and sustained exertion all require energetic support. When support capacity narrows sufficiently, the body often limits discretionary expenditure before more severe destabilization occurs.

Downshift therefore frequently represents intelligent allocation under strain rather than character failure.

This does not mean every reduction in motivation or function should automatically be normalized or ignored indefinitely. Persistent, severe, worsening, or unexplained reductions in function deserve appropriate attention rather than dismissal. The important distinction is interpretive. Reduced output under fatigue conditions does not automatically indicate laziness, weakness, or poor attitude simply because motivation declined.

The body may be protecting itself against escalating instability.

Importantly, downshift is not identical to total shutdown. Many people continue functioning partially during downshift states, but with narrower tolerance, slower recovery, reduced flexibility, and increased effort cost underneath ordinary activities. The system is still operating, though under increasingly constrained conditions.

This partial functioning often creates confusion because the person can still technically complete tasks under pressure when necessary. Observers may therefore assume adequate capacity remains intact. Physiologically, however, the body may simply be overriding reduced accessibility temporarily through additional activation while still carrying significant underlying strain.

The system remains constrained even when occasional output spikes occur.

This explains why some people can temporarily perform at high levels during emergencies or deadlines while collapsing afterward. Downshift reduced ordinary accessibility because sustained output had become too expensive. Acute activation temporarily bypassed the restriction. Once the activating condition ended, the underlying constraint became visible again, often more strongly than before.

The body had preserved continuity at additional cost.

Downshift also helps explain why emotional and social tolerance frequently narrow under fatigue conditions. Emotional regulation, conversation, empathy, conflict navigation, and sustained attentional engagement all require energetic resources. Under constrained conditions, the body reduces access to these expenditures partly to preserve remaining reserve for more essential functions.

The resulting withdrawal is often interpreted interpersonally rather than physiologically.

Again, the important distinction is not that every behavioral change is purely metabolic. Human experience remains psychologically and socially complex. The point is that reduced output accessibility often reflects physiological allocation under strain rather than moral failure alone.

The body continuously regulates how much function remains safely available under current conditions.

This understanding changes the meaning of fatigue substantially. Fatigue is no longer interpreted solely as low energy or lack of motivation. It becomes a regulatory language through which the system communicates strain, narrows expenditure, preserves reserve, and attempts to prevent deeper destabilization under rising load.

Downshift therefore is not defeat. It is the body reducing output to preserve stability when continuing at previous levels has become too expensive relative to available support capacity.

And when strain continues accumulating beyond the body's ability to preserve continuity through ordinary downshift alone, another threshold may begin emerging underneath fatigue itself. The system can eventually move from reduced output into broader functional disruption, where normal fatigue transitions into more significant instability across multiple layers of function simultaneously.

# Threshold Mechanism

Fatigue rarely emerges from a single moment in isolation. More often, strain accumulates gradually while the body continues absorbing demand through reserves, compensation, adaptation, and narrowing stability margins. Sleep loss may remain manageable temporarily. Stress may appear tolerable for a period of time. Fuel instability may produce intermittent discomfort without obvious disruption. Recovery debt may remain partially hidden beneath routine and obligation. The system continues functioning because buffers still exist between current demand and actual functional limits.

Eventually, however, the remaining reserve narrows enough that ordinary strain no longer stays contained smoothly.

At that point, fatigue frequently stops feeling merely uncomfortable and begins behaving more like functional disruption.

The Threshold Mechanism describes this directly: fatigue becomes functional disruption when accumulated strain exceeds the buffers and stability margins that normally absorb demand.

This distinction matters because threshold behavior explains why fatigue often appears sudden even after long periods of gradual accumulation. A person may tolerate rising strain for weeks or months while remaining relatively functional. Then, seemingly abruptly, ordinary tasks become disproportionately difficult. Concentration collapses more easily. Emotional tolerance narrows sharply. Recovery slows dramatically.

Crashes become more frequent. Small stressors feel overwhelming. Usable function declines rapidly.

The disruption appears sudden because the threshold crossing itself is sudden, even though the accumulation underneath it was gradual.

Human physiology depends heavily on buffers. The body continuously absorbs stress, instability, interrupted sleep, emotional demand, cognitive load, fuel variability, environmental strain, and adaptation pressure through multiple overlapping reserve systems. These reserves allow ordinary life to continue despite imperfect conditions.

Sleep reserve acts as one buffer. Recovery capacity acts as another. Fuel continuity, emotional regulation, nervous system flexibility, stress tolerance, electrolyte signal integrity, and broader metabolic stability margins all function similarly. These layers help prevent every single strain from immediately becoming visible fatigue.

Without buffers, ordinary life would feel continuously destabilizing.

The body therefore tolerates a remarkable amount of fluctuation before major disruption appears externally. A single poor night of sleep usually does not produce complete functional collapse because reserve capacity still exists elsewhere. One stressful week may feel difficult but still manageable because emotional tolerance and recovery systems continue absorbing load. A temporary period of glucose instability may create discomfort without immediately overwhelming usable function because broader capacity remains sufficient to compensate.

Threshold behavior emerges when these reserves narrow progressively across time.

The important point is that thresholds are dynamic rather than fixed. A demand that feels manageable under stable conditions may become disproportionately difficult once buffers narrow. The task itself may not have changed substantially. The system carrying it has changed.

This explains why ordinary demands often trigger fatigue disruption during periods of accumulated strain. The person may wonder why simple responsibilities suddenly feel overwhelming despite having managed far greater demands previously. Physiologically, the remaining reserve available to absorb those demands has been reduced progressively underneath the surface.

The threshold moved closer to ordinary life.

Compensation frequently delays recognition of this process. Earlier chapters described how caffeine, urgency, adrenaline, habit, routine, obligation, and activation can temporarily preserve visible output while underlying strain continues accumulating. During compensation, the body continues functioning through increasing regulatory expense. Fatigue signals remain partially masked because continuity remains prioritized.

This preserved output often creates the illusion that the system remains stable.

Underneath that apparent stability, however, reserves may be narrowing steadily. Sleep quality deteriorates. Recovery debt accumulates. Emotional tolerance decreases. Fuel continuity destabilizes. Nervous system activation remains elevated. Electrolyte coordination becomes less resilient. Stress load raises baseline operating cost continuously.

The body absorbs strain successfully until it no longer can do so comfortably within remaining margins.

Downshift frequently appears before full threshold crossing because the system attempts to reduce expenditure proactively as reserve narrows. Motivation decreases. Movement slows. Concentration shortens. Emotional engagement becomes more difficult. Social tolerance narrows. The body attempts to preserve stability through reduced output before deeper disruption occurs.

Threshold crossing occurs when even these protective reductions are no longer sufficient to contain accumulated strain smoothly.

This process helps explain why fatigue crashes often feel disproportionate relative to the final triggering event. The visible stressor immediately preceding the disruption may appear relatively small. A missed night of sleep, an argument, a deadline, travel, illness, emotional stress, heat exposure, or a demanding day may suddenly produce severe fatigue, fog, heaviness, or reduced function.

The final stressor was often not the sole cause.

It was simply the point where accumulated strain exceeded remaining buffer capacity.

This distinction removes much of the confusion surrounding delayed consequences. The body frequently appears functional during the accumulation phase because reserve systems continue compensating underneath ongoing load. Disruption appears later because thresholds depend on cumulative reserve depletion rather than on isolated events alone.

The resulting fatigue therefore feels abrupt even though the destabilization was building gradually for some time.

Stress load plays a major role in threshold behavior because sustained vigilance steadily increases baseline operating cost. The body reallocates resources continuously toward adaptation, prediction, emotional regulation, and continuity maintenance under prolonged uncertainty or pressure. This elevated operating expense narrows available reserve gradually even when outward performance remains relatively intact.

Ordinary demands then begin crossing thresholds more easily because the system possesses less unused capacity available to absorb them.

Recovery debt contributes similarly because incomplete restoration accumulates underneath visible functioning. A person may continue operating adequately while restoration repeatedly falls short of demand across time. The body slowly loses flexibility, reserve depth, and recovery efficiency underneath routine continuity.

Eventually the margin separating manageable strain from functional disruption becomes very small.

Fuel continuity also influences threshold behavior because unstable glucose availability increases regulation burden underneath ordinary activity. Crashes, fog, irritability, and unstable energy continuity reduce the body's ability to sustain smooth function under additional demand. Small fluctuations therefore produce larger consequences once reserve capacity narrows sufficiently.

Electrolyte signal integrity functions similarly. Signaling coordination, muscular responsiveness, circulation, and nervous system regulation all contribute to how effectively the body absorbs stress and maintains usable function. When communication quality becomes less stable, the threshold for disruption lowers because maintaining ordinary coordination consumes greater effort.

The body becomes more fragile under conditions that previously felt manageable.

Importantly, threshold crossing should not be interpreted catastrophically. Human physiology naturally operates through thresholds continuously. Temperature regulation uses thresholds. Hunger signaling uses thresholds. Sleep pressure uses thresholds. Emotional tolerance, muscular fatigue, concentration capacity, and recovery systems all behave similarly. The existence of limits is part of normal physiology rather than evidence of failure.

The problem is often interpretive rather than structural.

People frequently assume that because fatigue disruption appeared suddenly, the system must have failed suddenly. More often, the body had been carrying accumulating strain for an extended period while reserve systems continued containing it quietly underneath.

Threshold behavior simply makes the accumulated cost visible.

This also explains why fatigue tolerance fluctuates so dramatically across different periods of life. The same individual may handle intense demands relatively smoothly during one phase while struggling under ordinary demands during another. The difference often lies not in character, discipline, or willingness, but in available reserve and stability margin at that moment in time.

The body responds according to current support capacity rather than according to identity or expectation.

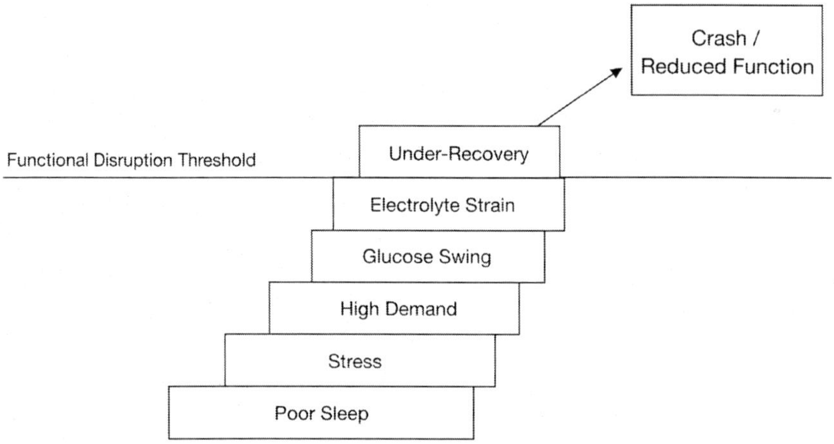


**[Figure 16: Fatigue Threshold Model]**

The relationship represented here clarifies why fatigue disruption often appears sudden after gradual accumulation. Small strain blocks such as poor sleep, stress, high demand, glucose swings, electrolyte strain, and under-recovery accumulate progressively underneath visible function. As these loads rise, reserve capacity and stability margins narrow quietly across time. Once the accumulated burden crosses the Functional Disruption Threshold, ordinary demand can no longer be absorbed smoothly, and fatigue shifts into more visible crash patterns or reduced function.

This framework changes how fatigue crashes are interpreted. The body is not suddenly becoming weak or irrational. The system has crossed a limit where available buffers are no longer sufficient to contain current demand comfortably.

Thresholds therefore represent system limits rather than character verdicts.

This distinction matters because many people internalize threshold crossing as personal failure. The sudden inability to sustain ordinary output feels emotionally confusing precisely because previous functioning may have remained intact for so long. The person remembers operating successfully under difficult conditions and assumes the present disruption must therefore reflect loss of discipline, resilience, or motivation.

Physiologically, however, the system may simply no longer possess enough reserve to continue absorbing strain invisibly.

The threshold became visible.

This understanding also helps explain why recovery after disruption is often slower than expected. Once buffers narrow substantially, rebuilding reserve takes time because the body must restore flexibility, continuity, signaling quality, fuel regulation, nervous system stability, and broader support capacity gradually rather than instantly.

The visible reduction in demand may occur faster than the internal rebuilding of reserve.

Threshold behavior also explains why ordinary tasks become disproportionately difficult during fatigue states. The task itself may remain objectively simple. What changed is the amount of remaining reserve available to absorb the energetic, emotional, cognitive, or regulatory cost required to complete it smoothly.

The body is operating closer to its current limits.

Importantly, threshold crossing is not the entire explanation for every fatigue pattern. Human physiology remains complex and layered. Persistent, severe, worsening, or unexplained disruption deserves appropriate attention rather than dismissal. The important point is interpretive clarity. Fatigue often behaves according to cumulative thresholds rather than isolated events.

The body continuously absorbs strain until remaining reserve narrows enough that ordinary demand can no longer be stabilized efficiently.

This perspective removes much of the moral language commonly attached to exhaustion. Thresholds are not evidence of weakness, laziness, fragility, or lack of character. They are expressions of capacity, reserve depth, regulation cost, and accumulated load across time.

Human physiology always operates within limits.

Fatigue becomes more understandable once those limits are viewed through stability margins rather than through personal judgment alone. The body continuously negotiates between demand, restoration, adaptation, and reserve preservation. When buffers narrow sufficiently, fatigue shifts from manageable strain into more visible disruption because the system can no longer absorb ordinary demand smoothly within its remaining capacity.

Thresholds therefore are not failures of effort. They are boundaries of available stability under accumulated strain.

And once threshold behavior becomes clearer, fatigue patterns themselves begin looking different. Temporary fatigue, recurring fatigue, crash cycles, fluctuating recovery, and gradual capacity drift can all be interpreted not as isolated events, but as evolving relationships between load, reserve, recovery, and the changing stability margins that determine how much strain the system can absorb across time.

# Fatigue Pattern Mechanism

Fatigue becomes easier to misunderstand when it is viewed as a single isolated sensation. One difficult day, one crash, one poor night of sleep, one period of heaviness, or one afternoon of low energy rarely explains very much by itself. Human physiology fluctuates continuously. Stress changes. Sleep varies. Fuel timing shifts. Emotional demand rises and falls. Activity changes across days and seasons. Temporary fatigue can emerge under completely ordinary conditions without necessarily indicating deeper instability.

Patterns become more meaningful than isolated moments.

The Fatigue Pattern Mechanism describes this directly: fatigue becomes more interpretable when its timing, recurrence, trigger context, recovery behavior, and drift across time are viewed as system patterns rather than isolated failures.

This distinction matters because fatigue is often interpreted emotionally rather than structurally. A person feels exhausted during a difficult afternoon and immediately assumes something is wrong with them personally. Another person experiences several weeks of gradually worsening heaviness and dismisses it entirely because no single moment appears dramatic enough to justify concern. Both interpretations mistake isolated sensations for the broader relationships shaping them across time.

The body rarely communicates through single events alone.

Human physiology behaves through patterns because regulation itself unfolds continuously. Sleep quality influences the following day.

Stress load accumulates gradually. Recovery debt compounds quietly underneath routine continuity. Glucose instability amplifies certain times of day more than others. Compensation delays visibility. Thresholds make accumulated strain appear sudden. Restoration lag causes fatigue to remain present after obvious demands have already decreased.

Fatigue therefore often becomes interpretable not through one sensation, but through recurrence, timing, drift, and relationship.

Temporary fatigue is the simplest pattern because it remains closely tied to a relatively clear stressor or demand. A difficult week, disrupted sleep, illness, travel, emotional strain, physical exertion, or concentrated cognitive demand may produce fatigue that resolves relatively proportionately once restoration improves and load decreases.

In these situations, the fatigue behaves more like an immediate response than a recurring system pattern.

Temporary fatigue still matters. The body is signaling real demand and real energetic cost. The important distinction is that the fatigue remains relatively contained rather than becoming chronically cyclical, progressively worsening, or increasingly disconnected from obvious triggers.

The body absorbs strain and then gradually restores capacity afterward.

Recurring fatigue behaves differently because timing itself begins carrying information. The exhaustion repeatedly appears under similar conditions, at similar times, or following similar forms of demand. Afternoon crashes emerge repeatedly. Morning heaviness becomes common. Post-meal fatigue appears predictably. Emotional stress repeatedly produces delayed exhaustion. Social interaction consistently narrows tolerance afterward.

The recurring nature of the fatigue reveals relationship rather than randomness.

This is important because recurring timing often exposes system strain more clearly than isolated intensity alone. A single afternoon crash may reveal little. Repeated crashes occurring after poor sleep, prolonged stress, delayed meals, or high cognitive demand suggest broader instability in energy continuity, recovery reserve, or stress regulation.

The body is not merely becoming tired randomly. It is revealing patterns in how demand interacts with current support capacity.

Morning fatigue illustrates this clearly. Some people experience the greatest heaviness immediately after waking rather than later in the day. The issue is not necessarily lack of sleep duration alone. Sleep-recovery translation, nervous system activation, restoration lag, stress load, glucose continuity, recovery debt, or ongoing immune strain may all influence whether sleep actually rebuilt sufficient capacity overnight.

The pattern itself becomes more informative than any single morning alone.

Afternoon drops often reflect different relationships. Fuel timing, stress accumulation, glucose variability, cognitive load, nervous system strain, and compensation fatigue may all contribute to declining usable function later in the day. Again, the goal is not certainty or self-diagnosis. The important shift is interpretive. Recurring timing frequently reveals system interactions more clearly than isolated exhaustion.

Post-meal fatigue can behave similarly. The body continuously coordinates fuel movement, insulin signaling, digestion, circulation, nervous system regulation, and energetic distribution after intake. Under strained conditions, these processes may produce heaviness, fog, reduced concentration, or narrowed tolerance following meals.

The fatigue pattern itself suggests that energetic coordination is interacting with current system state in meaningful ways.

Post-stressor fatigue reveals another important pattern. A person may feel relatively functional during periods of acute pressure only to become disproportionately exhausted afterward. Earlier chapters described compensation and restoration lag as important parts of this process. Stress activation preserves continuity temporarily. Once the stressor ends, the accumulated regulation cost becomes more visible.

The delayed timing often confuses interpretation because the fatigue appears after the demand rather than during it.

The body, however, frequently reveals accumulated strain only after immediate adaptation is no longer prioritized.

Crash cycles represent a more unstable fatigue pattern because usable function rises and falls repeatedly across time. Periods of temporary alertness alternate with crashes, fog, heaviness, irritability, reduced tolerance, or narrowed output. Compensation often contributes strongly here. Caffeine, urgency, adrenaline, obligation, and stress activation preserve output temporarily while recovery debt, glucose instability, and rising regulation cost continue accumulating underneath.

The body repeatedly exceeds its comfortable stability margin and then falls back into visible fatigue afterward.

Crash cycles therefore often reflect instability in continuity rather than stable low energy alone. The person temporarily functions above sustainable support capacity before the accumulated cost becomes difficult to continue suppressing. Fatigue then appears sharply until activation rises again and temporarily restores visible output.

This instability frequently feels emotionally confusing because the person alternates between feeling relatively functional and profoundly depleted.

Physiologically, the system may be oscillating between compensation and threshold crossing repeatedly.

Gradual capacity drift behaves differently from crash cycles because the change unfolds slowly enough that the person often adapts to it incrementally. Concentration becomes slightly more difficult across months. Recovery takes longer. Social tolerance narrows progressively. Physical heaviness increases gradually. Ordinary tasks require more effort than they once did. Sleep feels less restorative. Motivation becomes harder to sustain consistently.

No single moment appears dramatic, yet the baseline slowly changes.

This gradual drift often reflects accumulated recovery debt, rising regulation cost, persistent stress load, reduced adaptation reserve, narrowing stability margins, or unresolved restoration lag operating continuously underneath daily life.

The body slowly becomes more expensive to stabilize.

Because the progression is gradual, people frequently normalize the decline internally. They assume the exhaustion simply reflects personality, aging, weakness, or reduced discipline. The pattern itself, however, may reveal a broader systems relationship unfolding across time.

The body is continuously adapting to unresolved strain rather than simply failing randomly.

Importantly, pattern recognition should not become self-diagnosis. Human physiology is complex, and fatigue patterns alone cannot produce certainty about underlying causes. Persistent, severe, worsening, unusual, or unexplained fatigue should not be dismissed simply because patterns appear recognizable superficially.

The goal is interpretation rather than conclusion.

This distinction matters because many people move from confusion directly into rigid self-labeling. Every afternoon crash becomes assumed glucose dysfunction. Every period of heaviness becomes assumed hormonal failure. Every stress-related fatigue pattern becomes assumed nervous system collapse. These interpretations often oversimplify what are actually overlapping system relationships involving recovery debt, stress load, fuel continuity, compensation, sleep quality, threshold behavior, and broader support capacity.

Fatigue patterns are clues, not diagnoses.

The body communicates through recurring relationships because physiology itself is relational. Sleep influences stress tolerance. Stress alters fuel regulation. Fuel continuity affects concentration and emotional resilience. Compensation delays visibility. Thresholds create abrupt disruption after gradual accumulation. Electrolyte signal integrity shapes coordination quality. Recovery debt narrows reserve capacity across time.

Patterns emerge because systems interact continuously rather than operating independently.

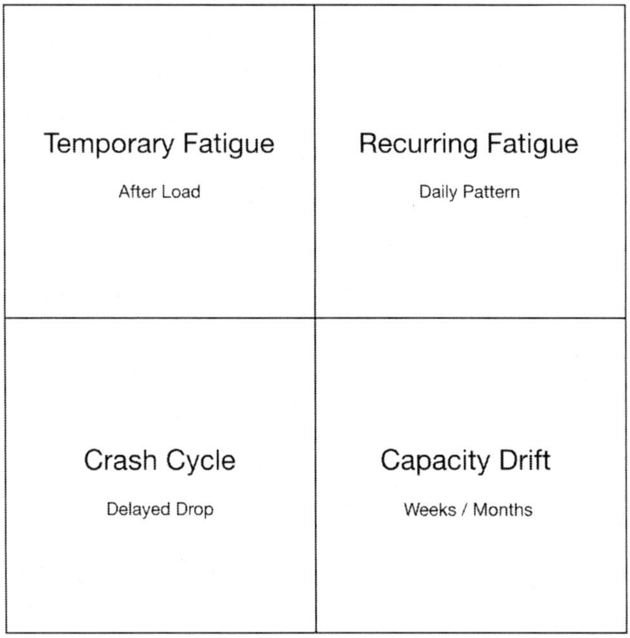


**[Figure 17: Fatigue Pattern Map]**

The relationships represented here clarify why fatigue becomes more interpretable through recurrence and timing rather than isolated moments alone. Temporary fatigue appears relatively close to the demand that produced it. Recurring fatigue follows recognizable timing relationships such as morning heaviness, afternoon drops, or post-meal exhaustion. Crash cycles involve repeated oscillation between temporary compensation and visible collapse. Capacity drift unfolds gradually across weeks or months through narrowing reserve and rising regulation cost. Each pattern reveals different relationships between load, recovery, fuel continuity, stress strain, and stability margin.

This framework changes how fatigue is interpreted emotionally. The body is not communicating moral failure through these patterns. It is revealing how demand, restoration, regulation, and reserve interact across time.

Timing itself often becomes physiologically meaningful.

This is why recurring fatigue patterns deserve calm interpretation rather than dismissal or panic. A single difficult day may simply reflect ordinary strain. Repeated timing relationships often reveal broader continuity problems underneath ongoing function. The body repeatedly encounters the same constraints under similar conditions because the underlying system relationships remain unresolved.

Again, this does not mean every recurring pattern indicates severe dysfunction. Human physiology naturally contains rhythms, fluctuations, and adaptive variability. The important shift is interpretive awareness. Fatigue becomes more understandable when viewed across recurrence, timing, triggers, recovery behavior, and gradual drift rather than through isolated emotional reactions to single episodes.

The body behaves through patterns because adaptation itself unfolds through time.

This perspective also helps explain why fatigue often feels inconsistent. Different mechanisms dominate under different conditions. Stress load may shape one pattern. Recovery debt may shape another. Glucose variability may sharpen certain crashes. Compensation may temporarily preserve output before delayed exhaustion appears. Threshold crossing may suddenly convert manageable strain into functional disruption after long periods of gradual accumulation.

The resulting experience therefore appears variable because the underlying system relationships are variable.

Pattern recognition helps organize this variability without oversimplifying it.

This removes much of the shame attached to recurring exhaustion. Fatigue patterns are not character verdicts. They are expressions of how the body is currently coordinating load, recovery, fuel continuity, regulation cost, nervous system strain, and broader stability capacity across time.

The body continuously reveals relationships through recurrence.

And once those relationships become visible, fatigue begins looking less like random weakness and more like an evolving map of system constraints interacting underneath ordinary life. The next layer of interpretation then becomes understanding which specific constraints are most likely shaping those patterns and why certain forms of strain repeatedly narrow usable capacity under particular conditions.

# Constraint Mapping Mechanism

Fatigue becomes easier to interpret once it is no longer viewed as one isolated sensation demanding one isolated explanation. Earlier chapters established that fatigue can emerge through multiple overlapping mechanisms involving recovery debt, stress load, fuel continuity, glucose variability, electrolyte signal integrity, compensation, threshold behavior, transition strain, and broader load-capacity mismatch. By this point, the important shift is no longer asking whether fatigue exists, but asking what kinds of constraints are most likely shaping the pattern being experienced.

This movement from sensation toward relationship is constraint mapping.

The Constraint Mapping Mechanism describes this directly: fatigue becomes more interpretable when patterns are mapped to likely constraint areas while preserving uncertainty and avoiding single-cause explanations.

The distinction between interpretation and diagnosis matters immediately here. Constraint mapping is not a process of assigning certainty to symptoms. It is not a self-diagnosis system, a medical triage framework, or a checklist for labeling every fatigue experience. Human physiology is too interconnected for fatigue patterns to reduce cleanly into rigid categories.

Constraint mapping instead asks a different question.

What kinds of system pressures appear most consistently related to the fatigue pattern being observed?

The body continuously communicates through timing, recurrence, trigger context, recovery behavior, threshold response, and drift across time. These relationships do not create certainty, but they often provide clues about which forms of strain may be narrowing stability margins most significantly.

Fatigue therefore becomes more interpretable when viewed relationally rather than morally.

Timing is one of the clearest starting points because fatigue patterns often behave differently depending on when they appear. Morning fatigue may suggest a different relationship than afternoon crashes. Post-meal heaviness differs from delayed post-stressor exhaustion. Gradual decline across months behaves differently from sudden instability after concentrated load.

The timing itself does not diagnose anything. It simply changes the probability landscape of which constraints may be interacting most strongly.

Morning fatigue, for example, often raises questions about sleep-recovery translation, nervous system downshift, restoration lag, ongoing stress activation, or unresolved recovery debt. The body may have spent time asleep without fully rebuilding support capacity underneath. Sleep duration alone may therefore reveal less than the relationship between sleep and restored function.

The fatigue pattern becomes informative not because morning heaviness proves one cause, but because the timing relationship repeatedly points toward overnight restoration dynamics.

Afternoon drops frequently suggest different interactions. Fuel timing, glucose continuity, accumulated stress load, cognitive depletion, compensation fatigue, or narrowing reserve may all contribute. Again, the point is not certainty. Afternoon fatigue does not automatically equal glucose dysfunction or nutritional failure. The body is simply revealing that usable function narrows repeatedly during a specific period of the day under recurring conditions.

The recurring timing becomes a system clue.

Post-meal fatigue introduces another type of relationship. Digestion, circulation, insulin signaling, nervous system regulation, and energetic redistribution all interact after intake. Under certain strained conditions, this transition may amplify heaviness, fog, reduced tolerance, or narrowed concentration. The important observation is not that meals are inherently problematic, but that the body repeatedly responds to specific transitions with reduced usable function.

The pattern points toward coordination strain occurring around energetic redistribution and regulation.

Post-stressor fatigue behaves differently again. A person may remain functional during periods of concentrated demand while crashing afterward once activation decreases. Earlier chapters described restoration lag and compensation as important contributors to this pattern. The body preserves output temporarily through urgency, stress signaling, obligation, and narrowed focus before accumulated regulation cost becomes visible afterward.

The delayed timing suggests that fatigue may be emerging through accumulated adaptation cost rather than immediate failure during the stressful event itself.

Gradual capacity drift reveals yet another relationship. Function narrows progressively across weeks or months rather than through dramatic crashes alone. Recovery takes longer. Emotional tolerance decreases gradually. Ordinary demands feel increasingly expensive. Sleep becomes less restorative. The body slowly loses reserve and flexibility across time.

This pattern often suggests accumulating recovery debt, rising utilization cost, chronic stress load, unresolved restoration gaps, narrowing stability margins, or broader load-capacity mismatch.

Again, these are probabilities rather than conclusions.

Trigger context provides another important layer of interpretation because fatigue rarely emerges independently from surrounding conditions. Stress exposure, poor sleep, delayed meals, emotional conflict, concentrated cognitive demand, illness, heat, social overload, disrupted routines, travel, or prolonged adaptation pressure all change how the body allocates resources and preserves stability.

Patterns become more meaningful when viewed in relation to these surrounding conditions.

Fatigue that repeatedly follows prolonged stress exposure may point toward elevated regulation cost, nervous system strain, restoration lag, or stress-driven glucose instability. Fatigue emerging during long gaps between meals may suggest constrained fuel continuity or transition strain. Fatigue intensified by poor sleep may reveal narrowing recovery reserve or impaired sleep-recovery translation. Fatigue worsening during heat exposure or prolonged sweating may suggest reduced fluid stability or electrolyte signaling strain.

None of these observations create certainty independently. The body rarely operates through isolated mechanisms.

This is why simplistic single-cause explanations distort fatigue interpretation so easily. Human beings naturally search for one answer because single-variable explanations feel emotionally satisfying. Everything becomes blamed on cortisol, carbohydrates, hydration, sleep, stress, hormones, or motivation individually.

Physiology behaves more relationally than that.

Stress load alters glucose regulation. Poor sleep increases compensation cost. Recovery debt narrows threshold reserve. Electrolyte instability amplifies muscular inefficiency. Fuel instability reduces emotional tolerance. Nervous system activation interferes with restoration depth. Compensation delays visibility while increasing future operating expense.

Fatigue patterns therefore usually reflect overlapping constraints interacting simultaneously.

Recovery response adds another important layer because the way fatigue changes after reduced demand often reveals as much as the fatigue itself. Temporary fatigue generally improves relatively proportionately once restoration increases and load decreases. Delayed fatigue may continue after the original stressor resolves because restoration lag remains active underneath. Recurring fatigue repeatedly returns under similar conditions because the underlying relationship remains unresolved.

Accumulating fatigue behaves differently again because reserve capacity continues narrowing despite temporary recovery attempts.

The recovery response therefore helps distinguish whether the body is handling strain temporarily, compensating repeatedly, drifting gradually, or approaching thresholds more frequently.

Recurrence strengthens interpretive clarity because repeated relationships generally reveal more than isolated events. One afternoon crash reveals relatively little. Repeated crashes following prolonged stress and delayed meals suggest stronger systemic reinforcement. One period of post-travel exhaustion may simply reflect temporary disruption. Recurring post-travel destabilization suggests narrower adaptability and reduced reserve flexibility.

The body communicates through repeated relationships because regulation itself is continuous.

Importantly, recurrence still does not create certainty. Persistent, severe, worsening, unusual, or unexplained fatigue should not be dismissed simply because patterns appear recognizable superficially. Constraint mapping is interpretive rather than diagnostic. It helps organize complexity without pretending the body behaves through perfectly isolated systems.

This distinction protects against overconfidence.

| | Fuel Access | Sleep / Recovery | Stress Load | Glucose Variability | Electrolyte Signal | Adaptation Cost |
|---|---|---|---|---|---|---|
| Timing | • | • | | • | | |
| Trigger | | | • | • | • | |
| Recovery Response | • | • | | | • | • |
| Recurrence | | | • | • | | • |

**[Figure 18: Constraint Mapping Grid]**

The relationships represented here clarify how fatigue becomes more interpretable through contextual mapping rather than isolated symptom labeling. Timing, trigger context, recovery response, and recurrence each interact with possible constraint areas such as fuel access, sleep and recovery quality, stress load, glucose variability, electrolyte signal integrity, and accumulated adaptation cost. No single pattern proves one isolated cause. Instead, recurring relationships gradually suggest which forms of strain may be contributing most strongly to the fatigue experience.

This framework changes how uncertainty itself is interpreted. Uncertainty is not failure of analysis. Human physiology is layered, overlapping, and adaptive. The body rarely presents fatigue through perfectly clean categories. Multiple constraints frequently coexist simultaneously.

A person carrying significant stress load may also have unstable sleep-recovery translation. Recovery debt may overlap with glucose variability. Compensation may conceal narrowing reserve. Electrolyte strain may amplify muscular heaviness underneath broader adaptation fatigue. Fuel continuity problems may worsen emotional tolerance while stress activation destabilizes energetic regulation further.

Constraint mapping therefore works probabilistically rather than absolutely.

The goal is not to eliminate ambiguity completely. The goal is to improve interpretive clarity enough that fatigue begins looking less random and less moralized. Patterns reveal relationships between demand, restoration, energetic continuity, nervous system regulation, stress burden, adaptation reserve, and broader support capacity.

The body becomes more understandable once these relationships are viewed together rather than separately.

This perspective also removes much of the shame attached to recurring exhaustion. Fatigue patterns are not character verdicts. They are system clues emerging from interacting constraints across time. The body continuously attempts to preserve continuity under changing conditions. Fatigue becomes visible when those conditions exceed current reserve, increase regulation cost, destabilize energetic continuity, or narrow recovery margins.

Constraint mapping therefore shifts the question away from "What is wrong with me?" and toward "What kinds of strain appear repeatedly connected to reduced stability?"

That shift preserves both humility and usefulness simultaneously.

It avoids simplistic certainty while still allowing meaningful interpretation. The body may not reveal one perfectly isolated explanation, but recurring relationships still matter. Timing matters. Trigger context matters. Recovery behavior matters. Threshold patterns matter. Drift matters. The interaction among these elements gradually reveals where support capacity may be narrowing most consistently.

And once these pressure points become more visible, another important shift begins emerging underneath fatigue interpretation itself. Stability improves not through one isolated correction, but through restoring coordination among load, recovery, fuel continuity, sleep quality, stress exposure, signal integrity, nervous system flexibility, and the broader support capacity required to sustain usable function across time.

# Stability Restoration Mechanism

Fatigue rarely improves through one isolated correction because fatigue itself rarely emerges from one isolated mechanism. Earlier chapters established that exhaustion can reflect output constraint, recovery debt, stress load, fuel instability, rising utilization cost, transition friction, sleep-recovery disruption, electrolyte signal strain, compensation, threshold behavior, and narrowing support capacity interacting across time. The body continuously coordinates these systems together rather than separately.

Restoration therefore behaves less like a single intervention and more like the gradual return of coordination across systems that had drifted out of alignment.

The Stability Restoration Mechanism describes this directly: fatigue becomes less dominant when the systems shaping load, recovery, fuel access, stress exposure, signal integrity, and capacity are brought back into better coordination.

This distinction matters because fatigue is often interpreted through simplistic correction models. A person searches for one missing variable, one dietary rule, one sleep target, one stress solution, one supplement, one hormonal explanation, or one behavioral adjustment that will suddenly eliminate exhaustion completely.

Human physiology rarely restores itself that way.

The body functions through relationships. Load interacts with recovery. Sleep quality influences glucose stability. Stress alters fuel continuity.

Nervous system activation affects restoration depth. Electrolyte signal integrity shapes muscular coordination and tolerance. Compensation masks strain temporarily while recovery debt accumulates underneath. Capacity narrows or rebuilds according to how these systems interact across time.

Fatigue therefore decreases most reliably when broader coordination improves rather than when one isolated variable changes alone.

This does not mean every mechanism contributes equally at every moment. Certain constraints may dominate under specific conditions. A person carrying severe sleep disruption may experience substantial instability through impaired recovery translation. Another may be more heavily influenced by prolonged stress activation or unstable fuel continuity. The important distinction is structural. The body restores stability relationally rather than mechanically.

The system improves through coordination.

Load reduction alone illustrates this clearly. Reducing visible demand may help decrease strain, but lower activity or fewer responsibilities do not automatically restore usable function if sleep remains fragmented, nervous system activation remains elevated, fuel continuity remains unstable, or recovery debt remains unresolved underneath. A person may technically "rest" while still carrying substantial regulation cost internally.

The body requires restoration depth, not merely reduced movement.

This distinction explains why passive rest sometimes feels insufficient after prolonged strain. The visible workload decreases, yet fatigue persists because deeper restoration processes remain incomplete. Sleep quality may still be poor. Stress signaling may remain elevated. Fuel stability may remain inconsistent. Emotional buffering may still require disproportionate effort. The nervous system may not have fully downshifted into restoration despite reduced external demand.

Reduced load and restored coordination are related, but they are not identical.

Recovery depth therefore matters more than surface rest alone. Human physiology restores capacity through layered processes involving sleep quality, nervous system downshift, energetic continuity, tissue restoration, immune recalibration, emotional regulation, and broader metabolic coordination. Time spent inactive does not automatically guarantee these processes are occurring efficiently.

The body may remain physiologically expensive to stabilize even while externally resting.

This is why sleep quality often matters more than simple sleep duration in fatigue restoration. Time asleep matters because it creates opportunity for recovery, but restoration depends on whether sleep actually translates into nervous system downshifting, reduced regulation cost, hormonal rhythm coordination, and support capacity rebuilding underneath.

The body restores itself through effective recovery translation rather than through unconsciousness alone.

Fuel access and glucose stability also influence restoration because usable function depends partly on coordinated energetic continuity across changing demands. The body requires reasonably stable access to fuel in order to preserve concentration, emotional tolerance, muscular coordination, and broader continuity throughout the day.

This does not mean perfect glucose flatness or rigid fuel control. Human physiology naturally fluctuates across feeding, fasting, activity, stress, and recovery conditions. The important point is smoother continuity rather than abrupt instability. When glucose availability becomes less volatile and fuel transitions become more coordinated, the body often spends less energy compensating for energetic disruption underneath ordinary function.

Regulation cost decreases when continuity improves.

Metabolic flexibility contributes here as well because smoother transitions between feeding states, fasting states, rest, activity, and changing demand reduce transition friction across systems. The body becomes more adaptable when fuel access and demand coordination remain relatively aligned.

Fatigue therefore often decreases not because the body eliminates fluctuation entirely, but because fluctuation becomes easier to absorb within broader stability margins.

Stress containment plays a similarly important role because prolonged activation dramatically increases operating cost underneath ordinary function. Earlier chapters established that vigilance, uncertainty, emotional suppression, adaptation pressure, and continuous nervous system activation consume resources even without visible physical exertion.

When stress signaling decreases appropriately and nervous system regulation becomes less continuously activated, the body spends fewer resources maintaining defensive coordination.

This reduction in regulation cost preserves more usable capacity for concentration, emotional tolerance, physical effort, and recovery itself.

Importantly, stress containment does not mean eliminating all stress from human life. Human physiology is adaptive and built to tolerate challenge. The issue is not the existence of demand, but whether activation remains continuously elevated without sufficient restoration depth and recovery flexibility afterward.

Stable systems are not systems without pressure. They are systems capable of moving between activation and restoration without becoming trapped in chronic regulatory expense.

Electrolyte signal integrity also contributes to restoration because coordinated signaling supports muscular function, circulation, nervous system communication, and broader system responsiveness. When fluid balance and signaling quality become more stable, the body often feels less heavy, less diffuse, and less effortful overall.

Again, this should not be reduced simplistically to intake rules or supplementation culture. The body regulates signaling quality through interacting relationships involving sleep, stress, activity demand, recovery state, circulation, fuel continuity, and broader physiological coordination.

The important shift is interpretive. Stable signaling reduces friction across systems.

As coordination improves, ordinary movement often feels smoother. Emotional buffering requires less effort. Physical tolerance broadens. Cognitive continuity stabilizes. The body spends less energy compensating for communication instability underneath ordinary function.

Capacity rebuilding emerges gradually from these interacting improvements rather than from one isolated correction alone.

This rebuilding is important because fatigue reduction is ultimately an output of restored support capacity rather than merely a direct target itself. Earlier chapters established that fatigue frequently represents protection, boundary enforcement, downshift, threshold signaling, compensation cost, or accumulated adaptation burden. The body increases fatigue visibility partly when continuing current output threatens broader stability.

Fatigue therefore decreases when the system has less reason to amplify warning or restrict output.

This perspective changes the meaning of restoration entirely. The goal is not perfect energy, permanent motivation, or uninterrupted productivity. Human physiology naturally fluctuates. All people experience temporary fatigue, periods of strain, and varying capacity across time. Stability does not mean eliminating every signal or every difficult day.

It means improving coordination enough that the body no longer needs to narrow function as aggressively or continuously in order to preserve stability.

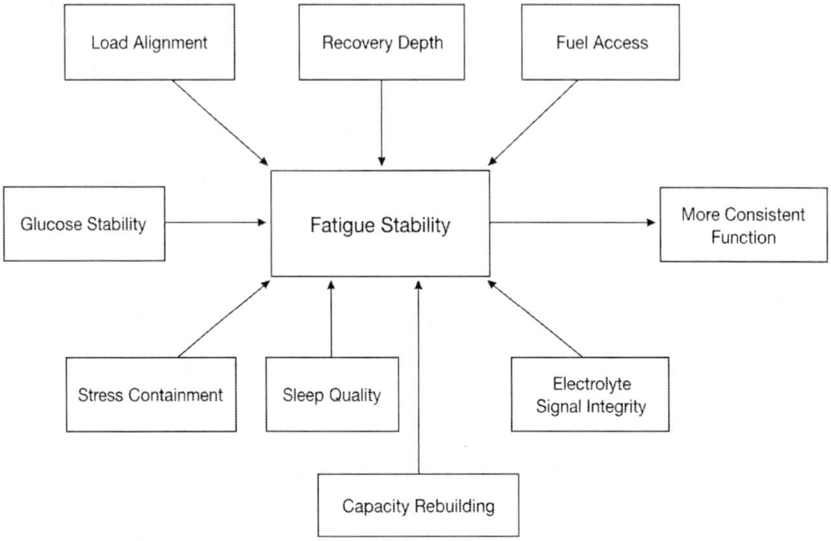


**[Figure 19: Stability Restoration System]**

The relationships represented here clarify why fatigue restoration emerges through coordination rather than isolated correction. Load alignment, recovery depth, fuel access, glucose stability, stress containment, sleep quality, electrolyte signal integrity, and capacity rebuilding all contribute interactively to broader fatigue stability. As these systems become more coordinated, regulation cost decreases and more consistent usable function becomes possible. Fatigue reduction emerges partly because the body no longer needs to enforce the same degree of warning, downshift, or output limitation.

This framework also explains why restoration often unfolds gradually rather than instantly. Human physiology rebuilds reserve through layered coordination across systems. Sleep quality may improve before emotional tolerance fully returns. Fuel continuity may stabilize before recovery debt fully resolves. Stress activation may decrease before nervous system flexibility completely rebuilds. Capacity restoration therefore unfolds progressively rather than through immediate reversal.

The body restores margins before it restores effortless function completely.

This gradual progression frequently frustrates people because visible demand may decrease faster than support capacity rebuilds underneath. Earlier chapters described restoration lag and threshold behavior as important parts of this process. The body often requires time to restore flexibility, reserve, signaling quality, and adaptation depth after prolonged strain.

Fatigue may therefore remain partially present while coordination improves incrementally underneath.

This does not mean restoration is failing. Human physiology rebuilds continuity gradually because recovery itself is an active process requiring coordination across multiple interacting systems.

Importantly, this chapter does not propose a universal solution or prescriptive formula. Persistent, severe, worsening, unusual, or unexplained fatigue should not be dismissed simply because certain patterns seem understandable conceptually. Human physiology remains complex, and significant fatigue deserves appropriate attention when necessary.

The important distinction is explanatory rather than diagnostic.

Fatigue becomes more understandable when viewed as a coordination issue rather than a moral issue. The body narrows output, increases heaviness, amplifies warning, reduces tolerance, or enforces downshift partly because maintaining stable function has become too expensive relative to available support capacity.

When coordination improves, the body often requires less protective signaling.

This understanding closes the central arc of fatigue stability. Fatigue is not merely low motivation, weak character, lack of discipline, or insufficient effort. It is a systems signal emerging from relationships among load, recovery, fuel continuity, stress regulation, signaling quality, nervous system flexibility, and broader support capacity across time.

The body continuously adjusts output according to how safely and efficiently it can sustain function under current conditions.

Fatigue therefore is not reduced primarily by defeating the signal itself. It becomes less dominant when the underlying coordination problems producing strain, instability, rising regulation cost, and narrowed reserve begin moving back toward greater alignment.

The body no longer needs to enforce the same degree of warning when stability margins improve.

This does not create permanent perfection or endless energy. Human systems remain dynamic, adaptive, and finite. Demand still exists. Fatigue still appears. Recovery still matters. Stress still alters capacity. Sleep still influences restoration. Fuel continuity still affects usable function. Human physiology continues fluctuating across time.

But fatigue becomes less disruptive when the body has less reason to protect itself through continuous downshift, amplified warning, or narrowed output.

And from this perspective, the meaning of fatigue itself begins changing fundamentally. Exhaustion stops looking like evidence of personal inadequacy and starts looking more clearly like information about system state, coordination pressure, reserve depth, and the ongoing relationship between demand and the body's current ability to sustain stable function across time.

# Fatigue as Information

Fatigue is often interpreted too quickly and too narrowly. A person feels exhausted, foggy, heavy, irritable, slow, unmotivated, or depleted, and the interpretation arrives almost immediately. The fatigue becomes laziness, weakness, poor discipline, low resilience, lack of drive, aging, failure, or personal inadequacy. The sensation is converted into judgment before the underlying system relationship is examined.

This book has approached fatigue differently.

Fatigue has been treated not as an enemy to defeat, but as information emerging from the relationship between demand and available capacity across time.

That distinction changes the meaning of exhaustion entirely.

Fatigue is not random. The body continuously regulates output according to available support capacity, recovery depth, energetic continuity, stress load, nervous system strain, sleep quality, fuel coordination, signaling integrity, adaptation reserve, and broader metabolic stability. Fatigue emerges partly when maintaining current function becomes increasingly expensive relative to available capacity.

The signal exists because the system is attempting to preserve continuity under strain.

This does not mean every episode of fatigue carries dramatic meaning. Human physiology naturally fluctuates. Temporary fatigue after concentrated demand is normal. Sleep disruption changes usable function. Emotional strain increases regulation cost. Travel, illness, heat, concentrated cognitive effort, social demand, recovery debt, and energetic instability all influence how much capacity remains available for ordinary function.

The important shift is interpretive rather than emotional.

Fatigue becomes more useful when it is understood as a systems relationship rather than a personal verdict.

This perspective removes much of the moral pressure commonly attached to exhaustion. Human beings often interpret reduced output as character failure because modern culture tends to value visible productivity more than physiological continuity. The body slows down, concentration narrows, emotional tolerance decreases, and ordinary tasks begin requiring disproportionate effort. The assumption becomes that greater discipline, greater willpower, or greater effort should override the signal indefinitely.

Physiology does not operate according to moral expectation.

The body continuously negotiates between demand and preservation. When strain rises faster than restoration, fatigue appears partly because the system is attempting to reduce destabilization cost. Recovery debt accumulates. Thresholds narrow. Stress load increases operating expense. Glucose instability disrupts energetic continuity. Compensation masks strain temporarily while reserve capacity decreases underneath. Sleep may no longer translate fully into restoration. Nervous system activation may remain elevated long after obvious stressors disappear.

Fatigue then becomes visible because sustaining previous output safely has become increasingly difficult.

The signal is protective before it is emotional.

This is why overriding fatigue indefinitely often increases system cost rather than resolving it. Compensation can preserve visible function temporarily through caffeine, urgency, adrenaline, obligation, habit, or stress activation. Output may continue for a period of time despite narrowing reserve underneath. But preserved output is not identical to restored capacity.

The body can continue functioning while simultaneously becoming more expensive to stabilize.

This distinction matters because visible productivity frequently hides rising physiological strain. Recovery debt accumulates quietly. Stress signaling remains elevated. Emotional buffering narrows. Fuel continuity destabilizes. Thresholds lower progressively. Fatigue signals may temporarily disappear beneath compensation only to reappear later with greater intensity once reserve capacity narrows further.

The delayed crash is often accumulated cost becoming visible.

At the same time, fatigue should not be dramatized or transformed into identity. The existence of fatigue does not automatically mean severe dysfunction, irreversible decline, or permanent instability. Human systems fluctuate continuously. Capacity changes across time. Demand changes across seasons of life. Stress exposure rises and falls. Sleep quality varies. Recovery reserve expands and narrows according to circumstance.

Fatigue is part of human physiology because adaptation itself has cost.

The goal therefore is not perfect energy or endless output. Stability does not mean the complete absence of fatigue signals. Stable systems still experience strain, temporary exhaustion, concentrated demand, and recovery periods. The difference is that stable systems preserve enough coordination and reserve to absorb ordinary fluctuations without prolonged destabilization.

Fatigue becomes more disruptive when strain repeatedly exceeds the body's ability to restore continuity underneath ongoing demand.

This is why fatigue belongs within the broader framework of metabolic stability rather than outside it. Energy continuity, glucose regulation, stress signaling, sleep-recovery translation, nervous system flexibility, electrolyte signal integrity, fuel access, adaptation reserve, and recovery capacity all interact continuously. Fatigue emerges partly through the interaction among these systems rather than through isolated failure inside one variable alone.

Human physiology is coordinated before it is compartmentalized.

The body continuously redistributes resources according to perceived need. Stress alters energetic allocation. Sleep quality changes restoration depth. Glucose variability influences emotional tolerance and concentration. Electrolyte signaling shapes coordination and muscular function. Recovery debt narrows available reserve. Compensation delays visibility while increasing future operating expense. Thresholds convert gradual accumulation into sudden disruption.

Fatigue becomes understandable once these relationships are viewed together rather than morally interpreted in isolation.

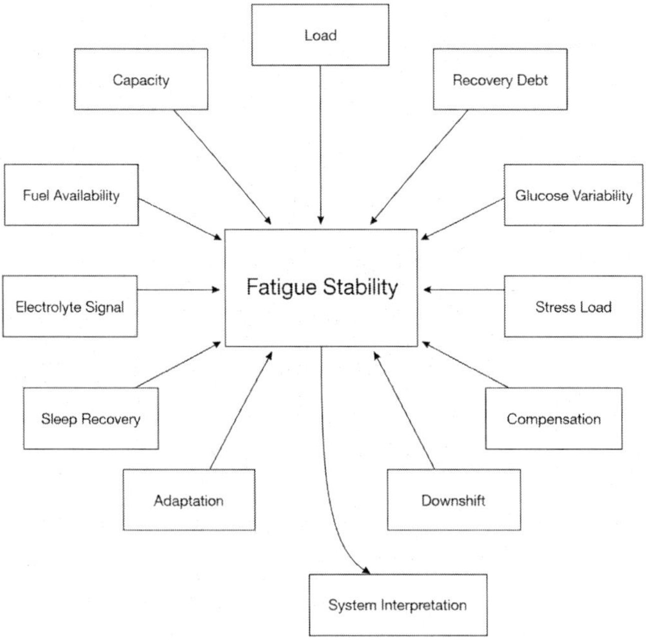


**[Figure 20: Fatigue Stability Integration Model]**

The relationships represented here clarify the full systems structure underlying fatigue stability. Load, capacity, recovery debt, fuel availability, glucose variability, electrolyte signal integrity, stress load, sleep recovery, compensation, adaptation, and downshift all interact continuously to shape fatigue expression across time. Fatigue stability emerges from the coordination among these systems rather than from one isolated variable alone. The feedback relationship between fatigue stability and system interpretation is especially important because how fatigue is interpreted influences whether strain becomes acknowledged, ignored, compensated for, or misunderstood.

Interpretation itself therefore becomes physiologically important.

When fatigue is treated purely as weakness, people often attempt to suppress the signal without understanding the conditions producing it. When fatigue is dramatized catastrophically, the signal becomes emotionally overwhelming and detached from structural interpretation. When fatigue becomes identity, every fluctuation feels permanent and absolute.

All three responses distort the signal.

The body is neither morally condemning nor emotionally attacking the individual through fatigue. It is communicating changing relationships between demand, support capacity, recovery depth, adaptation reserve, and broader physiological coordination.

Fatigue becomes useful when that communication is interpreted accurately.

This perspective also clarifies why stability restoration cannot be reduced to one correction or one explanation. Earlier chapters established that fatigue improves when systems move back toward coordination. Load becomes more manageable relative to available reserve. Recovery translates more effectively into restored capacity. Stress activation decreases appropriately. Fuel continuity stabilizes. Sleep quality supports restoration more efficiently. Signal integrity improves. Regulation cost decreases.

The body no longer requires the same degree of protective downshift or amplified warning.

Fatigue reduction therefore becomes an output of restored coordination rather than a direct conquest of the signal itself.

Importantly, this framework should never become an excuse to dismiss significant fatigue automatically. Persistent, severe, worsening, unusual, or unexplained exhaustion deserves appropriate attention rather than casual normalization. Human physiology is complex, and fatigue can exist within broader medical contexts that require careful evaluation.

The important distinction is interpretive humility.

Fatigue patterns reveal relationships, not certainty. Constraint mapping improves understanding without eliminating uncertainty completely. The body communicates through recurring patterns because physiology itself is continuous and relational. Timing matters. Recovery response matters. Stress exposure matters. Sleep quality matters. Fuel continuity matters. Compensation matters. Stability margins matter.

Fatigue becomes more interpretable when viewed through these relationships rather than through shame alone.

This final frame returns to the central idea that has shaped the entire book. Fatigue is not merely low motivation, poor character, weak discipline, or failure of effort. It is information emerging from the ongoing relationship between load and available capacity across time.

The body narrows output partly because maintaining continuity has become increasingly expensive under current conditions.

Misreading fatigue is therefore often more damaging than fatigue itself. When the signal is ignored indefinitely, regulation cost frequently rises further underneath continued strain. When the signal is moralized, interpretation becomes distorted by shame rather than guided by structure. When the signal is treated as identity, temporary physiological states begin feeling permanent and absolute.

Fatigue becomes most useful when it is understood as communication rather than condemnation.

The body continuously adjusts output according to current reserve, adaptation pressure, recovery depth, energetic continuity, and support capacity. Fatigue signals that those relationships require attention, not moral judgment.

And from this perspective, the meaning of exhaustion changes fundamentally. Fatigue is not proof of failure. It is information about the system. Stability begins when the signal is interpreted accurately.

**About the Author**

Nathan Reed writes about metabolic stability in systems exposed to load, variability, and time.

His work examines how biological capacity is shaped by energy availability, recovery architecture, sleep amplitude, muscle mass, environmental demand and workload. Rather than treating nutrition, fasting, sleep, and training as isolated tactics, he approaches them as interacting regulatory systems governed by margin, buffering, oscillatory coherence, and constraint dominance.

The Stability framework explores how physiological compression accumulates gradually and how proportional calibration preserves long-horizon resilience across decades. The objective is not peak optimization, but preservation of functional continuity under load.

Fatigue Stability is part of a broader metabolic stability ecosystem developed under Perennial Publishing, each volume addressing a distinct vector of biological durability.

The work is designed for readers who prefer structural clarity over motivational rhetoric and long-horizon coherence over short-term intensity.

**The Metabolic Stability Series**

Metabolic Stability – (Cornerstone Volume)

Fasting Fundamentals – (Foundational Volume)

Intermittent Fasting

Prolonged Fasting

Electrolytes

Insulin Stability

Glucose Stability

Metabolic Flexibility

Appetite Stability

Energy Stability

Blood Sugar Stability

Fat Loss Stability

**Fatigue Stability**

Future Titles Include:

The Vitality Series:

Sleep and Recovery

Strength and Aging

Hormones & Sexual Health

**Part of a Broader Stability Framework**

The Metabolic Stability Series is part of a larger stability ecosystem published by Perennial Publishing.

Related domains include:

Money Stability — structural durability in financial systems

Career Stability — positioning, load tolerance, and transition resilience

Mental Stability — cognitive steadiness under pressure and uncertainty

Emotional Stability — regulatory steadiness in environments that do not slow down

Foundations — low-fragility life architecture

Vitality — energy, strength, and biological function across time

Each domain approaches stability as a structural problem: capacity versus load, buffering versus shock, governance versus drift. Together, they form a unified framework for long-horizon durability across the major systems that shape human trajectory.

Made in United States
North Haven, CT
04 November 2026

21770476R00109